f[illegible] EVER [illegible] ENOUGH?

by:
Priti Kaur

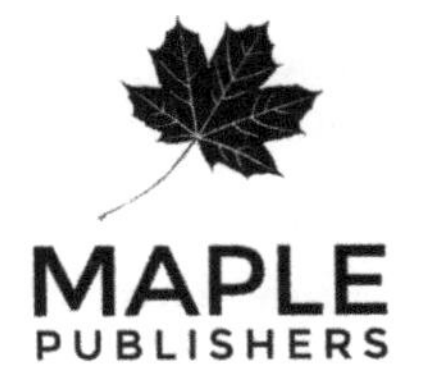

Am I Even Good Enough?

Author: Priti Kaur

First Published in 2023

ISBN 978-1-83538-078-9 (Paperback)
978-1-83538-079-6 (E-Book)

Book layout and cover designed by:
White Magic Studios
www.whitemagicstudios.co.uk

Published by:
Maple Publishers
Fairbourne Drive, Atterbury,
Milton Keynes,
MK10 9RG, UK
www.maplepublishers.com

A CIP catalogue record for this title is available from the British Library.

This book is a memoir. It reflects the author's recollections of experiences over time.

Contents

Dedication

This book is dedicated to my mother who is one of the strongest women I know on this planet. She has been through and sacrificed a lot to shape a better future for me.

Thank you, Mum, for always understanding and supporting me when my career choices have not gone as planned. Although at times you have passed judgment, I now understand through maturing it was because you only cared and worried for me. I love you and will always look up to you as my role model in life.

I hope my nieces and nephews grow up and learn that life is about making selective decisions. Whether or not they work out is a challenge and hurdle that will only make them stronger and work harder towards their chosen career path.

I do not want life to be simple because then how will we grow, learn, and teach life lessons to the next generation? My purpose in life is to educate others and to support them with my guidance and own life lessons.

Realising

Realisation has many definitions in the English dictionary but differs per individual due to their needs, wants, and situations. Realisation for me, means knowing something inside of me was always missing and after a few hurdles, I realised that I needed something that serves a purpose in life. I always knew it would never be easy and still, to this day, I continue to face these hurdles. But ask yourself, do you want to live your life for someone else or live it for yourself?

By profession, I am an ACCA Chartered Accountant which means I self-studied through my professional qualification by sitting fourteen exams followed by a few exemptions, an ethics module, and completing objectives. Why? - might you ask. This is because when I did apply for graduate schemes or roles that had study support packages, there were always too many requirements or as I will call it, box-ticking criteria that needed to be met.

After achieving a degree in Accounting and Finance (BA Hons.) from the University of Hertfordshire and achieving a 2.1 I thought I had done considerably well and made myself, but most importantly my parents, proud. I have always honoured my mum's approval. However, the route to success is never in a straight line and if you have achieved your success by being in the right place at the right time then one would say you are lucky. However, I had to face many rejections, opinions of others and mental health issues to finally secure a role.

The build-up to getting my first step in the world of Accountancy, involved me having to do an internship that did not help with finances that I would have used to invest in, myself, and it did not teach me any Finance-related tasks that I would need to secure a future paid role. The issue in today's society is that everything revolves around how qualified you are, what grades you achieved, and how confident you come across to an interviewer, but not everyone is the same. Sometimes the quiet ones are the hardest workers and the loud ones are the more sociable ones, but in essence, they both portray amazing qualities which are always transferrable and they will learn new skills during their life journey. It's important to always invest in yourself and do these courses to learn basic skills and then evolve them.

I will always be in favour of education. However, sometimes these qualifications we acquire never actually benefit what we need to do in reality in our day-to-day jobs; we have to acquire them to get a salary increase or a promotion. As I mentioned, I fully support education and I have gone through the process although I have learned some skills and knowledge which I have put into practice within my roles, but, essentially it is just a piece of paper that highlights that I have completed something. What it doesn't show is how many times I failed some exams, how I changed my exam techniques, how many hours I spent to achieve that certification and how much sleep I lost. Education is important but only if you then go on to learn from it and apply it in some way to your life; it is an investment in yourself and along the way even if you do not apply it to your day-to-day life, you will have learned other skills such as reading faster, organisation skills and other employable skills.

Nevertheless, I am glad I went through those emotions, stress, and studying because not only did I just begin my career but I also learned about the type of companies which appealed to me and what I wanted in return. For my part, I have always valued culture and flexibility in the roles I have undertaken. Have they all worked out? No. Am I okay with that being the case? Absolutely yes, because it only taught me what more I was seeking from a company.

When I landed my first paid Accounting Job, I was over the moon but also felt very scared, nervous and anxious because I had only just graduated from University and was looking for a paid study support package to help me to further my career. However, I did tell myself that it would not always be a straight-line journey. I worked in the transactional team as an accounting clerk which was not the most interesting role but I continued to build on my network in the company, talking with other Finance Teams and Managers to see where I could branch off to. I am not the most confident person when it comes to putting myself out there but a trial and error technique worked out.

I was then moved to another area in the transactional Team. The main reason for me wanting to move was simple. My previous manager was rude, unapproachable and always micro-managing me with ridiculous requests and workloads whereas my new manager, was very down to earth, willing to train me, and always helped me correct my mistakes so that I improved. She had taken a chance on me and it paid off because I remained in the company for a few years only because my manager made me feel valued and always supported me. I cannot stress enough how important it is to have the right manager, and one factor that everyone needs to consider before diving into a role just because it pays well or looks good on your resume. Yes, we need money to survive but your happiness and mental health come before your job and people, because when things go wrong, trust me when I say this, not everyone will support you. Some will worry about their issues over yours or just pretend like they never knew you were going through a hard time.

Those are the people we do not want in our life and if we do, they should be at an arm's length. Surround yourself with those who motivate you, inspire you, and remind you that it's okay to be yourself regardless of how ridiculous you may look; do not judge yourself on your history and the reputation that has been labelled to you. If people judge you, they have a shallow mindset or just do not deserve to get to know you more. You do not need to explain yourself to anyone, change yourself to meet their expectation, or prove you are worthy to be in their circle. Be you, you are good enough for yourself, you are the leader of your world and you will go through many life experiences to become wiser.

After learning the lesson of self-worth, I decided that over the years of working at this company, I needed a change and something more challenging, but this was only one of the very few reasons I left. The company went through a re-structuring and new employees were hired, some of whom were not competent to carry the tasks at hand, but that being said, I was always cordial and vocal with seniors about any changes I believe that were needed and why.

You cannot hire people for just filling a role, you should hire people who have a passion and show motivation to want to learn the role, instead, individuals were hired based on them being friends with senior management or previous experience of working with them. Although that is not an issue in itself, it becomes an issue when they leave after a few months because they do not know what they are getting themselves into or they have a negative impact on the team due to their lack of motivation and desire to help the team.

With the above being said, it led me to question the integrity and culture of the company. There was an upcoming role for an Accounting Manager which was discussed with me. I was in the position to get this. However, after being pulled into a meeting room with the Head of Finance, I was told that individuals had mentioned that I was too vocal about the running of my team. Although this was a shock to me, the role was given to someone else, based on favouritism. Companies will find any excuse to throw you under the bus and to excuse themselves from a promise they have previously made. I was upset by this but I did not show my emotions in the meeting because no matter what I said or did, it would be overlooked or ignored. There was no point defending myself. Even though I had asked who had mentioned this, they were not able to state names or recall what I had said that was truly offensive. After reflecting upon this, I realised I had been vocal with my Manager, away from the open platform in a formal professional manner. Was I rude about my thoughts and feedback? No. But I was transparent in changes I believed were needed to allow a more efficient way of working.

However, like most hiring companies this was often ignored, or I was told it would be discussed later.This is something you expect when you work with individuals who only care about profit, meeting deadlines, and making a status for themselves. Eventually, with me being vocal, I was labelled as being involved in company politics. Well, if voicing my opinion formally and professionally away from the open platform is making me look negative then, clearly, I do not belong in a place that has a top-down approach. If our leaders in the Finance function are asking us to be open with seniors in catch-ups or one-to-one then I am in my right to do so. Why act like a role model to only then be a hypocrite? We are often told to be ourselves at work and to treat people how we want to be treated. Let's be honest, how true is that? You cannot be yourself at work, you have to be a fake version of yourself to please people, you have to be a 'yes' person because if you say 'no', it leads to other consequences and you have to always have your guard up because there are always a handful of people who try to drag you down or try to overstep you to show they are more deserving of your position.

Requesting something from your employees is just as important as listening to their views because who knows, they might have a great idea or something that is not being picked up due to seniors being too focused on attending meetings that add no value. One thing that I have taken away from my experience here was that management had a narrow tunnel vision approach and they were not willing to invest in my ACCA studies although I asked many times as I had passed the probation period. Also, they were not willing to help me grow within the company or offer a promotion once I had proved my abilities to my committed role. They were more invested in promoting others whom they favoured, who, needless to say, had never worked in my team or had any previous knowledge.

The point I am trying to make here is, companies need to review their mission statements and values. If you say you encourage and promote something then practise what you preach, let employees know that it is okay to speak freely and that their job will not be at stake. We are all trying to survive and earn an income, so why do a handful of us always try to bring others down? bYou do not earn any credit for it so why spend so much energy to do it? Our role in life is to not entertain the bullshit but to attack it back with kindness because we are complex humans, we have personal issues, internal pressures as well as external pressures, but one thing, we are not cruel individuals trying to make a statement about others' productivity, standards of work or how slow someone is.

If someone is struggling, talk to them, they may be going through mental health issues or something more personal outside of work. I ask you, readers, that if you see someone having a hard time just show empathy and try to support them or give a helping hand for a while. We all have bills, families and goals so unite to help one another because all you are doing is increasing the profit for the CEO or founder of the company but you are not taking any of that profit.

On a positive note, happy days were to come as after months of applying for other roles or signing up with recruitment agencies, I secured a role with a company in a different industry, which was well recognised worldwide. Again, this did not come easy. I had been told by many recruiters before I even secured this role that I was not experienced enough or I had too many exams left to sit to complete my qualifying accounting title and after months of crying, feeling depressed and having panic attacks I never gave up on myself.

There is one particular memory that runs through my mind as a constant reminder. I remember meeting a start-up recruitment agency in Central London, who after twenty minutes of meeting me, gave up on me and told me to come back to them after I had established myself more. I then walked back to the station but on my way there I stood on the side of the street and cried my eyes out and called my mum and said I wasn't good enough. Another rejection, what am I going to do with my life? It's been over four years and even now I look back and think I wish those recruiters could see how I have built myself up from scratch and how I never lost hope.

The lesson I took away from this was, I will never let anyone tell me that I am not good enough or that I cannot do it; dreams can become a reality if you work on your mental state and pitch yourself well but also if organisations take chances on people. End of the day we are all humans and we all have our financial duties but investing in someone who doesn't tick all the boxes will not only be you doing a good deed, but you are making a difference in someone's life, you need to put yourself in their shoes. We all have struggles which are covered by fake smiles.

Have an open mind and be willing to try and understand the person you are interviewing rather than judging them based on their resume. Even if someone meets fifty percent of what you are looking for then it's enough. Meetings can always repeated or moved unless there are strict hard-core deadlines for compliance, then those are excused. But from a high-level point of view, time should be taken to invest in those who are ambitious and show the right attitude; there is enough time during work hours to prioritise needs and wants.

However, despite these rejections, when I did get a new job and the opportunity to work with some amazing clients, it was very overwhelming. The office was huge, beautiful, and very corporate, which was breath-taking, weirdly, but for the most part, my team was amazing. The woman who interviewed me was very humble, direct, and approachable, and that was a huge bonus for me as we had similar personalities and began a friendship outside of work. Whilst working on the contracted client in my role for a few months, I got to travel to different sites and meet more stakeholders.

This was the most enjoyable part of the job as I always took it upon myself to use this as a learning curve. I learned how to adapt my tone and body language towards certain people, whom to trust and be outspoken with, when to be a good listener but more importantly I never let anyone feel small or not valued. Some of the junior staff in the role who reported back to me felt undervalued and overworked but I always assured them that they were the backbone of the operations and the true success to the company's revenue.

No matter how small the role or what hierarchy someone fits into, they are the backbone to the foundation and should always be treated with respect and given recognition and praise. Praising or calling out a team is not hard work, and if anything only requires a few seconds. Communication and respecting individuals are overlooked in modern society. We live in a world of emails and messages where any misunderstandings can be avoided through individuals simply calling one another and having more of an interactive approach.

This also in my experience gets any expectations clear and avoids any miscommunication as questions can be asked directly. This technique works very well and has been tested by myself and I can promise you that the results produced after are amazing, and more time effective rather than wasting time going back and forth via emails.

On the other hand, whilst I was being a small motivational speaker for my team, I became very invested in the team, tasks, and individuals' needs and wants. One issue is that those who are junior do not understand why they do the tasks they do and how they contribute to the bigger picture or the company's role. The message is often, we need this report by this time, when will you be able to get this across. This is the very exact issue that starts the hierarchy status because you are not valuing your staff, you are not explaining why you need the information and how it will be used to be presented to wider departments but furthermore, the true workers behind the reports do not get credited or recognised as it's always rewarded to the presenter.

Your work will be handed over to someone else to use as their starting point, who will then go and develop it further with some fancy graphs and charts and then take the credit. This demoralises staff and reduces their productivity. This is the issue that we all have faced in one way or another in our careers and if you have not, it is yet to come, but this experience should be taken in your stride; it will only make you learn more about what you want from a company's culture and what you will do differently once you reach a higher position. We often learn from our leaders and follow in their footsteps as we idolise them and assume they are successful because of how they portray themselves or act, but you are wrong.

You need to seek what you want to be as a leader. Yes, you can copy some skills from your leaders and adjust them to suit your style but furthermore, you need to show your personality. When you become the leader and then go on to teach others, always remember where you once were, and if you ever forget, just take a moment to put yourself in their shoes and reflect on it for five minutes. Reflection is key to being successful as well as being open to criticism because not only do you grow as a person but you learn how to improve your skills further.

One benefit of me starting back at the bottom of my career in this new company was not only that I got paid more than in my previous role but I had a mentor who taught me the ropes and always explained to me why I was doing certain tasks and then how they contributed to the reports and statistics projects which were to be presented to the senior management team who would be relying on our information to design the budgets and forecasts.

What I took away from this was how to then go and explain this to the juniors and ensure they understood their tasks. After they completed their tasks, I would then go on-site, to show them how I used their information and numbers to create reports and how they would be presented to others in the team. Not only that, but I was also involved in meetings where I was able to listen to ongoing changes in the contracts, new reports needed, and how performance was going.

This was so beneficial as I was able to learn the same information as my seniors which allowed me to be more productive, generate ideas, and be ready for what was to come in the future and ensure that I was prepared. This is one thing that is often not done in corporations, so new information comes as a shock or surprise to employees or they have less time to prepare themselves for tight deadlines or last-minute adjustments to files.

Imagine if the culture was more open and transparent in the office, juniors would be more efficient, feel valued, and feel empowered to experience as though they contributed to the success of a task or project. If a company is going to be open and transparent, you need to be able to listen to your employees and allow them to speak freely in an informal manner and present any ideas and concerns. In the same vein, these need to be respected and actioned accordingly. Office life is about teamwork and not about sitting behind your desk and producing report after report.

If this is the case why are you going to the office? Organisations need to embrace a culture of honesty, no judgment, no stupid ideas, but stability, and involvement.

Whilst I had all these working in my favour, unfortunately, we lost the contract, and therefore my only options were to either TUPE over which means moving across to the new bidding company, or to find another contract within the company. My last resort was leaving and starting somewhere new, but the social pressure we receive from recruiters about how a short role looks bad on my resume, considering I had been in the role for less than six months or so, gave me severe anxiety. However, I acted like this did not bother me when in fact I started feeling worthless and depressed.

I went for an interview with the company that had now won the bid and was offered a role as a Finance Manager which at first, I thought was a big leap in my career but the responsibilities were not compensated in the pay. Usually, when it comes to a role I enjoy, I want to be comfortable, with managed stress and know that I will learn something from the role. If I feel these personal wants are met then I do not consider money as my number one factor, but, you need to find the balance and consider your standard of living. I knew the money was not good but I would learn so much more than I had ever imagined.

Where there is a rainbow, there is always a storm to follow. Once again, I felt like the world was against me. I was told that the role was no longer open and I was made redundant. I couldn't even explain how my soul just left my body. I thought to myself, I did everything right, moved jobs to get more exposure and once again I am stuck and told I am not good enough. I just wanted the world to work in my favour for once and to give me some hope. I applied for roles internally and my team put out a good word for me about my work ethic and helped me build some connections but once again I was not good enough to get recognised or seen as an asset.

I had done one of the ACCA exams whilst in the role and thought this would surely show them that I could balance my work and education and still stay late to complete tasks very close to exam week. Everything I did during my time in the role was me just trying to show my worth because let's face it, sometimes it's about who you know rather than what you know.

Even though I cried for days and days, it came to my final week on the contract. I was in communication with HR regarding my P45 and leaving package when suddenly my Finance Team Lead told me that they had a new role in a new contract that they had just landed. He asked if I would be interested in meeting one of the Finance Managers who was managing one of the Regions. I jumped at the opportunity and had my first team call with her. My thoughts were, she seemed very nice and supportive, and was very keen to help me learn more technical finance techniques which would benefit my exams.

I was super happy and pitched myself for the role. Furthermore, she knew who I was as I volunteered to try tests of a new system that was going to be launched in the future and had to report back on features and functionality. She admired my enthusiasm and personality, which again goes back to my point of branching yourself out so you create a rapport with people because you will be remembered if you portray yourself as an asset. Just like everything in life, it's about creating your brand. It may not always work but that does not mean you let bad experiences ruin your mindset to try it again.

I was then offered the role in the new team and contract which would be operating globally. This meant I got to go around Europe for training and meet my operational and finance team in the countries under my portfolio. It's a dream that I thought I would never be able to achieve in a lifetime but working in a Finance role where I got to travel was just a mind-blowing experience. All flights and expenses were reimbursed and whenever we had a spare moment, I got to see a little of each country's culture.

I finally felt like I had found my dream role but to keep my place I still had a long way to go. Even though you are taught debits and credits and how to balance a statement of financial position nothing compared to what it was like doing it in an actual working environment. My manager was based abroad so it was difficult to always be trained or be able to contact her as she was busy with calls. Even if I did receive a call it was always rushed or time allocated on teams. Therefore, whenever she came to London I would stay behind late till ten in the evening or sometimes twelve in the early morning to learn how debits and credits worked in a working environment. My first task was Month-end. Even though I knew what it was and it sounded fancy, I had never seen it done.

My first training was my manager making me open a journal template and explaining to me what each button does, and how to upload and post. She would write the debits and credits on a piece of paper and then give it to me to type into the system-generated template and post, and then download the Profit and Loss account as well the balance sheet to see what changes were made. Even though this sounded so manual, I began to see a pattern of what accruals and prepayments were, why they were a debit or credit, and how double entry worked. We did this for a few days and completed Month-end. It was very draining due to the long nights. I knew it would get easier as I took more ownership.

As months went by I learned Excel formulas and was able to carry out my month-end journals, posting and presenting them to my manager and the Finance managers under my portfolio in each country. Any hurdles I faced, I reflected upon and became more proficient in my role. This was a light bulb moment for me as usually accountants do one month-end for their company but I was doing three to four month-ends in one week, with a worksheet showing my calculations and then making packs to present to seniors before the system locked. This became a repetitive monthly task.

Even though I owe a lot to my manager for teaching me the tasks and training me, the hours never seemed to slow down or become a routine nine to five. I realised that I was working over twelve hours a day, on my weekends, and sometimes offline during my annual leave. I was also messaged during my annual leave for requests. Being new to the field I thought this was normal and it was fine to graft for a few years as it would pay off.

Eventually, the travelling got draining, the long hours made me less productive, I became more irritated at smaller things, I felt hot-headed and I was not eating or sleeping properly. In essence, I felt like a Zombie who was on auto-pilot and just working but I was not able to engage in conversation or focus for long periods.

It got to a point where I began to resent my job and I began to doubt my career choice. I would often speak about this to my family and friends and I am sure they got fed up with me moaning but not doing anything. My mother would force me to eat or log off, however I knew if I did not complete a task it would affect the team or I would get in trouble or portrayed as not being a team player. I began to overthink, the doubts became worse, and I felt overly tired when eventually I collapsed.

I noticed that I suddenly found it hard to wake up but I would not listen to my body as I was determined to be the best version of me. What I never asked myself was, does being the best mean I need to work like a dog and sacrifice my health and well-being? Although I did mention to my manager - how long will this go on in the contract? The answer was simple. The contract is new so it will take a while for it to set up and become self-efficient. It had been a year now and things were still not better. The contract was just understaffed and people were overworked. It took me a while to realise this and even though I did not want to leave my role, the culture became too toxic, company politics were non-stop and everyone was out to get one another. I know that sounds like I am exaggerating but it is one of the employment opportunities I will never return to.

You need to always reflect on what you want from the role, and, is it enough for you? Suffering in silence and assuming things will get better is you being delusional. Some of you may enjoy and thrive on working late, feeling important and in power, and assuming you have to do it as a must. But is it a must or are you doing it because you think the consequences of you not doing the task will cause blame to be shifted to you? I can go on and on about the possible thoughts a person would have and how sometimes, as I say, we let our imagination run wild.

Even though I am thankful for the growth I had and how much I learned in a short space of time, I learned that if I did not learn to focus on my social life or my health then eventually down the line I would become very sick and, if anything, become someone that I don't even recognise anymore, let alone those who know me become distant. I needed to find a work-life balance and again, I only learned that through the journey I went on. I don't have regrets but I wish I was more vocal about my health being impacted.

I am sure by now I might have come across as someone who runs away if something doesn't work in my favour or the way I planned. It is fine if you are reading this thinking this very thought. However the difference is I know how important I am and how I need to listen to my body and thoughts. If you keep on going the way you are in a very fast-paced job which causes you to have no social life or always feel tired then you will regret it when you are older. I am thirty and I may be young but I have had it rough from the beginning so the world can no longer be a scary place, there are no more surprises that can make me feel low or unwanted. I have been there and learned from it. You are your number one priority and you are worth so much more if you open your heart and head to new possibilities. You might not see them straight away but life always has a meaning behind the signs it shows, find them and solve them. You will be amazed when you look back at what you have achieved, and take a leap of faith.

If someone does not achieve a first in their degree or have first time passes and seems shy in the interview, it does not matter because they will learn and adapt to the company culture if a chance is given to them. Talent slips away if you only pick the top individuals because they may be academically smart but do those grades and marks mean that someone will understand the role, duties and perform it well?

I hope that this book achieves its purpose of making companies revisit their talent requirements. Life is currently very hard with the cost of living increasing, mental health becoming a real issue and people becoming homeless. Everyone just needs a chance or hope that they will make it to their goal with smart working as opposed to hard working but it will come with sacrifices and we have to be willing to make them. If life was too easy then I would have been a millionaire by now.

Similarly, I have three siblings who all have amazing careers in Engineering, HR, and Logistics. They all seem like they know their end goal and what they want to achieve from their careers, but I always question why do I not feel the same way or are they hiding how they feel? The truth is, not everyone is as open and honest about how they feel or find it hard to put into words and just continue to follow the circle of life which is eat, work, sleep, and repeat.

But I always knew that circle of life and how we just follow our elders or how the system which is in place doesn't fit into my world. If anything, it made me more depressed, sad, and anxious about how I am going to continue the next fifty years like this. Do I just need to work to have a pension and some company benefits? Is that what life's purpose is? I refuse to accept this way of living.

As I said before I am an Accountant by trade so all my feelings, feedback and tips are all from my very own experience and this does not mean that my book only relates to accountants, females, or those who are lost. My life goal and aim are to help individuals realise their worth, feel confident to try new things even if they do not work out, and never give up hope based on the opinions of others. If changes are made or I have made someone think more deeply about their life choices then that is enough for me.

Delusional

Being delusional is a type of serious mental illness called psychosis in which a person cannot tell what is real from what is imagined. Delusional for me means believing that the way I was treated was correct and it wasn't real, and I was creating these mini-scenarios in my mind that seemed worse than reality.

After leaving my previous company, I became unemployed for a month or so where I signed up with recruitment agencies and started to research different roles that were out there in Finance. This was something that I needed to be open to because I have always been placed in roles that I thought were necessary for me to build a brand for myself and to make myself stand out to new employers or recruiters. The market is saturated, so you are given the impression that you need to stand out and be the best of the best against others. Although this is true in some form it also makes you believe that you need to be working every hour of the day or keeping yourself busy.

The lesson here is to work on one thing at a time. We worry too much about what is going to happen if we don't achieve or have X, Y, and Z completed to show on our resumes. However, ask yourself, do you want to keep worrying about what is going to happen in ten, or twenty years down the line? For all we know, we might not be here in this world. There is no guarantee that we might live to see tomorrow and as harsh as that sounds, we have enough problems to deal with on a day-to-day basis. When we think about problems that may arise but have not even happened, yet we create unnecessary stress, anxiety, and scenarios in our mind of what may or is going to happen when we simply do not know. Live life in the moment and take it a day at a time when things become hard. There is no expectation to create pressure of what we need to become.

This is exactly what I did. I decided that through applying directly for roles, I was not getting a response quickly enough or that I would never hear back. Once I signed up with a few recruitment agencies and updated my resume on Indeed and Reed more recruiters began to contact me. LinkedIn was the most beneficial one for me as I was able to see who the recruiter was, the job role, and what they desired in an individual. Did I tick all their boxes? No, but these were desirable things as opposed to essentials and therefore I decided that I may be given a chance to have at least a first-stage interview.

After weeks of trying and patiently waiting, as that is all I could have done, I was invited to some interviews. At this point, these were jobs that I found on LinkedIn. The first stage was discussing the role with the recruiter and then progressing on to booking an interview. The issue here was that most recruiters themselves did not know much about their client or the job role which was shocking as you are meant to be the promoter. Even though some recruiters were not helpful at all, I decided to go to the interview and do a lot of background research myself. I began to understand what the company does, its values, annual reports, and reading reviews on Glassdoor or other websites. This gave me an indication of what type of company I may potentially be working for.

One thing I would say is, do not jump into a role just because you need one as there are other means of support if it is needed, which I will go into in later chapters. If you attend an interview and know in your heart and head that it does not sound like the job ad which you applied for, then do not push for a second stage. If you are interested in hearing more and having the opportunity to ask further questions to clear your doubts and fears then attend the second interview. Ask questions, do not be an okay person and believe everything at face value, and believe that the questions in your mind will be answered on the job or after you secure the role. It may be late by then. You might not like the job at all. Therefore I encourage you to ask lots of questions and tailor them to ensure you get the answer that you want and always be sceptical.

If you have no doubts and believe it is the right role for you, give it a chance as after all, you have taken all the necessary steps to ensure that it fits your goals and desires. If you are unsuccessful then it's okay, be open to accepting feedback and reflect on it. You do not need to believe it is all true, but you need to be able to find a fine line of identifying how and why you got that feedback. Reflection is key because if you are delusional and believe you are too good for the employer, then you are not opening yourself up to grow. We all have negative thoughts when we are rejected and it's fine to have them for a while, but that time should be used to reflect on how you are going to tackle your next interview better and what extra preparation you will need to do. Don't waste that energy burning inside of you, use it as motivation and let your flames burn bright.

I, myself have been through the whole process. I have rejected some roles due to them being falsely advertised or the interviewers not fitting the personality or needs I want from my future manager. This was not about passing judgment, but it was the first impressions. If no one is smiling or inspiring you by explaining how amazing this job opportunity may be then it sets the tone that either that individual does not fit into your personality circle or that the culture is very much purely work-related as opposed to staff welfare. First impressions count and are important. If something does not feel right then trust your gut, you have lived through life and have had enough experience to know when something is not for you.

Other reasons I have left jobs is due to recruiters just being too pushy and making me feel very uncomfortable. This is just one instance that I have always reflected upon and in a way felt blessed that I had experienced it as it now taught me what to expect from a recruiter. This one recruiter never really understood the role they were meant to be managing or what their client company did. So, when I would ask questions, the answer was, to ask at the interview. When I would ask what the salary band or potential growth from other individuals they have placed in the role has been, the answer was that salary is dependent on the individual and how they come across and other individuals have grown in the company after two years.

It got worse. He would always book my interviews for the next day saying that was the only availability the client had, which was utter nonsense. I felt pressured and rushed to a point where I did not feel ready or relaxed to portray myself well. He would call me straight after my interview to ask me what questions were asked and how they reacted to my answers. Now at this stage, I did not understand why it was important for me to tell a recruiter because they should know more than me when they get signed up to represent a client.

However, only within the last year or two, I have realised that the recruiter wanted to know this information so that he could go and pass it on to other candidates in his portfolio. This has made me realise that some, not all, recruiters are just very keen to ensure that their candidates get selected so that they have a nice commission at the end and secure future roles to be represented by them. However, everyone should be given a fair opportunity to secure a role.

Furthermore, from my own experiences, I have had recruiters disclose how other candidates did and tell me what questions they were asked and how I needed to answer them. I do not want to give a scripted answer, I want to portray myself as who I am and not what I am meant to be. This made me think if all recruiters are the same. Am I wasting my time applying for a job and should I trust recruiters if they ever discuss a role with me? It was hard for me to accept that recruiters would even be useful to me.

I remained open-minded and eventually met some very good recruiters, but, as I mentioned, you need to be able to go through these hard battles of having poor experiences versus good experiences. This one recruiter is someone I have used for years and remained in contact with. Even though I may not be seeking roles at selective periods in my life, it is good to always remind them you are still present. He always listened to my wants and needs and ensured that he only put forward roles that fit what I was looking for. Even if the role ticks fifty percent of my needs I was happy because it's a compromise you need to make.

After a month or two of seeking a new role, I finally had an interview with a company that was the competitor of my previous employer. What a small world, I said to myself. The interview was with the direct hiring manager and even though the job only ticked fifty percent of what I was looking for, the hiring manager was the main reason I accepted the role. The interview went smoothly, and the conversation was flowing which told me that she would be very well to work with and she would also be someone I can look up to as she has grown in the company herself. I was offered the role the very same day and I accepted it.

The first three months of the role were very difficult for me as I set myself very early goals, in which I said I wanted to be a Finance Manager in eighteen months. Although it is good to have goals, we need to be realistic about them. Just because someone else might have got to your ideal position within that timeframe or even shorter, it does not mean the same will happen to you. You should always try to adapt and understand your role within the first three months and then set your goals from there with monthly or quarterly goals so that they are not too far into the future because this causes uncertainty. If you set yourself goals; for example, one of my goals was to be able to complete the first set of balance sheets and month-end within three or four months of me within the role, then make sure you are able to track your progress against this or understand why it was not met to learn from it.

Although this was achievable because I had previous technical experience, I just needed to learn how this company operated. What I will say is if you do not meet your goals, it's not the end. Just move it back a month or two to a point you know you can realistically achieve them. If this means having discussions with your managers or others to know the outcome of this being achievable then do so, do not set goals that disappoint or make you lose motivation. This is a skill that we all need to master.

Taking my advice, I began to overcome the fear of having to be the best. This was struck by previous experiences, whichare not always easy to forget as it does change us as a person. My manager was very understanding in that she expected it to take me three to six months to get a grasp of how things operated which made me feel more relaxed. From reflection, this was one of the best jobs I have had and an experience I cherish very close to my heart. Not saying that it was all roses because every role has its downfalls, but the pros overlooked this. I did stay in the role for just under two years as I was given more responsibilities, pay raises, and nominated for an award. The culture, my team, and my work-life balance were just perfect. I did work late for month-end but that was only for three or four days during the month for me to have my work up to date. It was never a requirement from my manager. This was something I admired because feeling valued made my output of work more efficient and made me enjoy the job a lot, to the point, that I wanted to work an extra few hours here and there. Sometimes the time would go so fast because I would get very invested in the work.

I am an individual who likes to be challenged and one who likes to learn new things whether that is financial systems or process changes. I was asked if I wanted to focus on a new portfolio, in a different division. This would have been a new challenge for me as I had no experience of how this division worked. It was also something that was completely out of my comfort zone. I would have to learn new systems, meet a new team, be the one person who was solely responsible for the month-end, and explain the results to seniors.

I started having delusional thoughts that the new team hated me, no one was supporting me, and I was not good enough or smart enough compared to the person who previously did this role. But these thoughts were all in my head, they were not real. The team did not have a chance to know me and understand how I liked to work but vice versa I never put myself out there to introduce myself to talk to the team or understand what each team member did.

My first thoughts were, shall I accept the role, even though I was offered it and I had a little briefing of the team and how the division operated, but did I want to move to a more complex part of the business? Another thought I had was why not let the new person who was joining our team, do this role, and then I could just grow within my current role with the hopes of being promoted. However, this was me being delusional. Was this going to happen, who knows? But I was certain it would. Again, I was doing those very things I had taught myself not to do, which was assuming situations in my mind.

After having discussions with my Manager, I decided that I would give it a go and it would not be fair for someone new to the company to work on a hard complex division. The current Manager of this division (my trainer) got in touch with me to discuss a schedule of the handover and the timeline this needed to be completed. We were currently in January, so I was given till March to learn the whole process of how the division worked, what reports I needed to use, how to generate them as well as other processes. I had not even started this new role within the company, and I already felt very overwhelmed. In January, my first task was to watch my trainer do month-end. We were constantly on calls for a few days where I watched how month-end was conducted and wrote notes. However, due to her having done the role for a few years, she was going too fast, and it was very hard to keep up. I instantly regretted my decision to accept the new challenge but thought I was not going to judge it straight away.

After we had completed month-end, I had to learn how to present the work and results in professional reporting templates and slideshows. Again, she rushed through this without explaining why it was needed. I felt myself becoming very irritated at this point. Once all those tasks were finished, I was told that she would email the files over to me so that I could play around with them and start understanding how the whole process works. However, yes, I would learn how the files would work and how I needed to tailor my reports and working files for different managers but it did not teach me why we were accounting for certain transactions in a certain way.

I thought it would be best to ask her if she had any previous notes that I could use as a training manual, but to my surprise the answer was 'no'. Well, this takes me to my next point. Yes, you are expected to learn on the job, but every company should have notes of processes recorded and stored for a rainy day. Let us imagine if someone is off sick and something important is needed, then it would be ideal to have these step-by-step notes with snips or screenshots to be readily available. Yes, this sounds manual but it's a one-off task that may need to be updated in the future, but the initial hard work would have been done at the beginning. However, as mentioned this was not the scenario in my case.

To make things worse, I was sent requests from my trainer to take action on certain tasks. There was not much information in the body of the email, the language in which the email was written was not to my understanding. This was because this certain division used lots of abbreviations and different words to refer to something. This alone was another challenge for me.

I decided that I needed to discuss this with my manager and the head of my new division before things got unpleasant. I mentioned that I was not being trained properly, nor time was being allocated for efficient training. There were no review notes, and I was being asked to take action on things that I had never done before. My manager was empathetic towards me but told me to take control and make it work for me.

I decided when it came to February's month-end that I would just need to be vocal about how fast the training was and how it was not working out for me. I told my trainer to allow me to do month-end with her giving me step-by-step guidance. I also took it upon myself to make a recording of the whole session on my phone and then to watch it back and make my own notes with step-by-step guidance and screenshots. I also did this as I did not want the person after me to struggle like I did.

Even though this was very time-consuming I knew I could have no reason to say I did not do all I could to make the transition into the new role work for me and I did just that. You must sometimes in life take things upon yourself and make yourself the expert. Furthermore, you need to establish what type of learner you are. Do you learn visually or like trying the tasks with someone guiding you or just being left alone to figure it out? I learned very early in my career that I was not a visual learner. I physically needed to try the tasks by having control of the mouse and screen in front of me with someone talking me through the steps I needed to take. This only needs to be done once or twice for me to get the bigger picture of the tasks.

When the February month-end was complete I did not hear anything from my trainer. She began to ignore my emails, always being on calls and not training me any further. I then decided that I was not going to keep on chasing for the training as I was not going to take responsibility for something seniors should be organising. Furthermore, it was just added stress which should not have fallen upon me. You need to know when to find the balance to stop taking everything upon yourself because you will just burn out. I learned that. I was just going to inform my manager and let her deal with getting the handover complete because I knew already that I had taken all the steps I could and now I was not going to allow the company to put me under even more pressure.

The month of March had come, and it came to me as no surprise that my trainer had been told that she needed to focus on her new role and that I would have to do month-end by myself. I was not able to ask my manager for help as she did not know how that division worked nor did she attend the training sessions with me, so everything was resting on my head. I put on a brave face and just watched the video I could of the previous month's end I recorded and kept resuming and pausing to ensure I captured every step correctly. Some things made no sense to me, but I decided to do the bulk of it and worry about the smaller things later.

The head of my new division was not a very kind or well-articulated man. He was often stressed, and this was evident through his tone and pace of speech; this did not help the situation at all. In fact, he was shocked that I even took a video of the whole session and was impressed that I thought of this idea, but he did not praise me as I was in the dark about a lot of other things. I worked four long days with six hours of sleep each day during the whole Month-end process. This is another experience I will never forget but it's one in which I have learned how to react if I ever had to give a handover to someone.

This is exactly what happened. After months of the head of my new division asking me to constantly change the budget or my workings files, I decided that he did not have a clue about what was going on in the contract. It became quite frustrating. It hit a peak point for me when we had a meeting with the client team who were very harsh in the month-end review. Instead of the head of my new division explaining and supporting my accounting decisions, which were done within the compliance and contract guidelines, he stayed on the call quietly and did not speak to support me.

He then sent an email to my manager stating that the meeting did not go well at all and that he had no clue how month-end was done. Even though I was fuming at this point as he had seen the month-end results prior to this meeting and had agreed it was okay, it came as a complete shock to me that suddenly, he was acting oblivious. There was nothing wrong with the work I had done but the client wanted it presented differently, going forward, which was not passed on to me.

I did not have a great relationship with the Head of my new division after this day and even though I was told to not reply to the email as by nature I am a reactive person, which is something I am working on, I did reply with my view of how the meeting went and how I felt very disappointed that someone that senior did not step up and live up to their job title. You would expect someone senior to speak up on your behalf when you feel attacked and then professionally speak with you one-on-one if they believed there was any miscommunication which led to the client team becoming confused. However, in my case, I will accept blame if I honestly feel it was an error on my end. In this case, the message was not communicated to me, and therefore rested with the Head to explain this to the client. However, we must remain professional, so I agreed to rework the slides and send them in a manner they preferred before the end of the day. This just created duplicate work.

What I am trying to get across here is that it is very important to communicate with your team no matter what the hierarchy status is. I have always loved a bottom-up approach as it creates a more inclusive culture. You will always fear that someone more senior than you knowsmore or is an expert in everything but they are not. They have life experiences and you may know more than them on certain topics, so do not be afraid to speak up and make suggestions. Do not assume anything or be in the unknown of thinking you are over-stepping your pay grade because if you limit yourself then you are shying away from showing your knowledge and interests in certain areas. Furthermore, I saw the benefits of this situation which was - I did not want to adopt those leadership qualities which he had failed to fulfil as the Head of the division. Therefore, I cannot stress enough how important it is to see negative or not-so-pleasant situations work to your advantage because, in these bad situations, you will only learn how to grow and what not to do. This is something you cannot just teach yourself; you must experience this whether it's in a job, in life, or personal situations with friends and family.

After a few months of covering the new division, I decided I was unable to work with the Head of this division and I was okay with making this decision for my own sanity. I decided I would look for another role before leaving and that is exactly what I did. Once I signed the contract for the new job, I resigned. I trained my colleague who was going to take over my role in a way I would have preferred to be trained, sent him all my notes, and let him conduct month-end with me guiding him face to face. Even after I left, I would always answer his call and help him out or explain things and this is because we built that connection and I knew what he was going through as I had experienced it myself first hand. It is always good to help others regardless of how you feel about others in the team and what you went through. You should not think from the point of view that I was treated this way so someone else should have it the same, they cannot have it easy. If this is the type of person you want to be then unfortunately it saddens me because you have not learnt the power of having great connections.

If you have knowledge then share it as it will not impact you in any way but if anything, it's a skill you are learning as you will be training someone; this is highly valued in organisations. What we fail to see is that everything we do is a skill we are learning. Even though it may not seem that way now, you will reflect on it when asked in interviews about your key skills. This moment right now is a skill you are practising, which is reading and being able to allow yourself to think and apply some of the things you have learned from these two chapters so far into goals and changes you want to make to your future life. Writing this book is also a skill for me and I have learned how to articulate my thoughts to get my messages across directly.

After one year and seven months of service within the organisation, I took away many lessons; one was focusing on the positives and always remembering what I had learned on the job. I even went as far as writing down all the positive and negative experiences, which I then reflected upon. This was because I wanted to start my new job being an even better version of myself. You must be open to keep on learning and pushing yourself to take risks. Do not sit in silence and do what I did in the past which is believing that something will get better itself. No, you need to make it better for yourself or have your voice heard to ensure the change happens. If it doesn't then take a risk and move on to focus on something which gives you true happiness even if that means taking a break from work as a whole.

This world is a scary place and it is getting harder so sometimes I understand you feel vulnerable, scared, or confused but that is life. You need to learn to always find motivation when you feel these emotions and just let nature take its course. I have always believed that when signs present themselves, they should not be ignored, they should be given deep thought and investigation to get to the root of why you feel a certain way, and this is the first step of growing as you learn to be self-aware. The second step to growing is reflecting on what things did not go as you planned and trying to understand it. Things could have been done differently to get the results you wanted. This will happen from time to time in life but learn from it and do it differently next time. The third part of growing is accepting criticism and the last step is not limiting yourself. There are a thousand opportunities out there so don't niche yourself because you do not need to fit into one box, you can branch yourself out. It will always be hard to get to the starting line but once you take those first steps you have completed the hardest challenge life can throw at you.

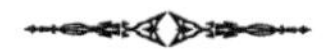

Mental Health

Mental Health is defined as a person's condition regarding their psychological and emotional well-being. Mental Health for me is defined as finding it hard to cope with my thoughts, feelings, and state of mind. Mental Health is something that has now become very serious in the world we live in; it has been around for years but only since the pandemic individuals have realised how common mental ill-health is. In some shape or form, we all suffer from mental health problems, we have low days, we have phases in life, and it's ok, but we need to remember to be kind and not to overlook those who just need someone to talk to. Even though we may find it hard to open up, it does not mean someone else will.

I, for one, have always suffered from anxiety and depression but I have never known the root cause. I got anxious when it was exam sessions at university, public speaking, or starting a new job. All of this is something we will experience if we truly care about something because it becomes a personal pressure to achieve those grades or goals you have been working towards. However, I started to notice that my anxiety got severely worse over the years, and I started having depressing thoughts. Even though I am not one to put myself out there, I did start to speak about my feelings and thoughts to my partner because he has always been the one person I can talk to openly about anything in the world. I find it harder to talk about these issues with my family as I find it hard to open up or often feel that I am going to worry them. I began to bottle up my feelings and ignore them when essentially, I came to a point of my life where I started having suicidal thoughts and began to self-harm myself.

I always knew in my heart that I needed to see a therapist who was professionally qualified to diagnose me and help me work through my issues. However, I could not find the courage to seek help as I thought I would come across as weak. I have always cared about my reputation and how I am portrayed in the eyes of others and now that I am older and wiser, I do not know why I cared so much because that only made it worse. I could have felt better a long time ago if I focused on myself. Another pressure was that I did not want my family to know that I needed professional help because this is not something that is openly discussed in my household.

The self-harming only occurred when I felt very low, angry, or like I had disappointed myself. Sometimes the pain felt sensational, and it turned into a habit. The colour of my blood, the marks, and the pain I felt when the water hit; it started to feel like a sense of release and even though the marks are now fading away on my arms and legs, it is always a reminder of how far I have come. I do not regret self-harming myself because at that moment in my life I just felt lonely and lost and the external pressures of who I was to be and how I was meant to act became overbearing, and regretting it will not make the marks disappear. My family was not aware that I was doing this to myself in my room or the shower and then crying myself to sleep. I have always felt like the black sheep of my family because they saw the world differently from how I did. They just followed the path of life whereas I was always questioning my way through life, but this caused me to feel as if I did not belong in the world and I would not cope if this was the way of living.

As I got older and began to stop self-harming myself, I found other means to cope, none of which were helpful. During University I discovered that I had alopecia, which is when you get bald patches in your hair. That was one of the toughest times of my life. Imagine being a student with bald patches on your head and being afraid that anyone behind you in the lecture room or the library can see it. I got so paranoid that I began to style my hair differently and placed lots of clips in my hair so if the wind blew, my hair was secure. The insecurity and voices in my mind drove me to distance myself from people and isolate myself. I would avoid social meet-ups or going out much because I knew if someone saw a girl with a bald patch then I would be labelled as ugly. These thoughts were all in my mind.

Negative thoughts tend to get worse if you keep on overthinking and dwelling on situations. However, me being me, I would think about problems that have not even occurred or exist which led to me having a lack of sleep and lack of appetite for years. This is something I have been battling for years. Only two years ago I got alopecia again but this time, I embraced it instead of letting it consume me. I knew I needed to change. I still have a lot of growing and healing to do and always will, because that is our purpose in life, to experience situations and learn from them.

Since the pandemic, I have now realised that I do suffer from mental health issues and I noticed symptoms of depression, social withdrawal, extreme feelings of pleasure, anger, mood swings, confusion, and others. If you can relate to any of these then allow yourself to seek help or work through each of your symptoms to understand why you feel the way you do, what caused it and what small initial steps will you take to work through them. It's important to note that this transition has no timeline, do not add that pressure to yourself, and work at a pace in which you feel comfortable.

This is something that I still need to work towards and one issue I have realised about myself is that I have never taken the time to just figure myself out and truly know who I am. I have always kept myself busy with employment. I have always been one who has had no gaps in my resume because I liked to have security but little did I know that you cannot run away from your problems and ignore them because, eventually, you will collapse.

Whilst I had left my last job to move to a more senior role in a new industry, it was a new challenge and one which I thought would be the right move for me. However, this role was hybrid and more than an hour's drive away from my home. This was a challenge for me because, in my previous role, I worked at home for the whole year and seven months, with odd visits to the client's site. Working remotely became a norm for me and one which I enjoyed due to saving time and money on travelling, being in the comfort zone of my home, and having no disruptions. However, the downfalls were, that at times I left lonely, missed human interaction and communication was slower, so I thought this hybrid model would be the best of both worlds.

I began my new job during summer and it only lasted four months as I voluntarily left. The reasons for leaving were due to me being bullied by my manager. My manager was a young chap, he had recently been promoted to Finance Manager and had been in the role for a few months. There was no doubt that he was very smart, and he was an Excel wizard, he was very confident in speaking with seniors, a quick problem solver, and knew how to please people. He was in his element but what he lacked was management, leadership, and people skills. It is very important to be able to lead your team and to be able to help them grow and be patient especially when they have entered a new industry like me.

The culture in this industry was very different from what I was used to. It was very fast-paced, deadline after deadline, and constantly changing. Furthermore, the role I applied for, was nothing like my previous job, there was not much comparison, so when I did secure the role, I was shocked that I even got selected. However, if they chose me, then clearly, they saw something in me or my skill set, linking back to my point about taking a leap of faith. The interview process itself was not difficult and included three stages but the on-boarding was terrible. As a senior, my role was to focus on the budget for all our stores, track daily sales, and discuss any anomalies. However, this company had new systems I had never used. Their spreadsheets were very manual with no workings showing how they derived those numbers, and it was very hard to be able to learn from previous people's work.

During my first week, I was told to book meetings with a handful of employees who had been in my position once upon a time or those whom I would be working very closely with. Furthermore, I must complete online training and play around with the system to get used to it, all of which are normal processes you expect during your first week of work.

The team was built up of graduates who were all on graduate schemes or some who had qualified years ago and got promoted within the company. The structure of the company was based on rotation which meant that you could apply for a role in another team after eighteen or twenty-four months but most of the time rotations were discussed in talent views bi-annually where the seniors of different finance departments would discuss who will be rotated or moved.To be considered you needed to tick a lot of appraisals and goals set by your manager, some of which as we all know seem as if we are doing a bit too much for the position, we are in. Then again organisations will maximize their staff instead of hiring additional support, which in turn leads people to leave. If it means going over and beyond in your role will teach you new skills, then embrace that extra mile of hard work.

I noticed that all the graduates and other members of the team had a very strong bond, due to them all having gone through the same process. As a new person to the team, you would expect to feel included and welcomed but most of the time I was left to sit there on my own and just quietly work on tasks that were never well explained. Again, my manager forgot that I was not used to the vocabulary, acronyms or style of reporting in this industry. I hated my first two weeks of the role; the team would go to lunch together and never invite me which led to me having my lunch in my car or just not eating at all due to how I was feeling. I decided that I needed to put myself out there or make the first move to be noticed.

As two weeks went by, I began to talk to the juniors, asking about their weekend, and joining in their conversations which worked for a while as I was able to ask for help but again was never invited for lunch. I began to see that the culture here was about finding a group and sticking to them and you could see that every day when everyone would sit in the canteen with their little group.

I had weekly one-to-ones with my manager; this was a time for me to discuss any concerns or worries and those thirty minutes were for me as opposed for my manager. I did mention that I felt very uncomfortable as I felt very excluded from the team and just felt as if I was not part of one and this was making me anxious. He did note this and began to invite me to lunch and made it arecurring habit during my team. He was unaware of this happening and agreed that it was not correct to be made to feel that way. However, that did not last long.

During my third week, I came in with a different mind-set. I was told that I needed to be in the office two or three days a week which I abided by and worked the remaining from home. I was given my first big assignment; this was emailed to me by my manager with little information about what I was meant to do. I was told that I needed to look at the previous examples from the lady in the role before me and recreate them for the upcoming year, which would be used to feed into the budget. Again, I am new, the spreadsheet was manual with all formulas hard-coded so there was not much I could have done. I wanted to show my strengths and decided to study the spreadsheet in the evening as well as write any questions or acronyms that I did not understand to be discussed in my next one-to-one.

When it came to my next one-to-one, I was given new tasks and deadlines which my manager explained to me briefly and then told me to have a go. Now, when you are in my position as a Senior, yes, you are expected to hit the ground running and be able to make spreadsheets work in your favour. This is something which I have enjoyed; I like to follow the same process but make the spreadsheets in a style or presentational form I prefer, and I am confident in explaining. This was allowed in this company. My previous employers on the other hand have had the same process for years which are strict hard templates that have to be used for compliance.

However, the point here is that you cannot expect a new starter to get started in a role with no clear explanations of what results you expected from the tasks, or to work through an example, explaining the worksheet, especially as I mentioned it is a new industry, role and first time seeing this requested task. No matter how junior or senior you are, this level of support should be given.

The issue is that sometimes Managers forget how to break things down or to be empathetic and this links back to my point of them treating others the way they were trained. Well, everyone has come from different backgrounds, different training styles, and different working environments so it doesn't mean because it worked for him, it would work for me. Furthermore, I was still learning how the industry operated and how the company as a whole was run.

Whilst I had completed a few smaller tasks myself which were then reviewed and returned to me to make any smaller changes, the feedback was always harsh or negative. I had only been in the role for a month at this point. As I had previously mentioned it is good to receive criticism and feedback from your seniors, but it needs to be constructive and well explained so that you can take learning points away from those reviews and then work on them.

In my case, my manager would discuss the smallest things such as font size, the colour of content, or rounding numbers, which was very tedious and something which did not require my work to be sent back and forth. This is something that a good manager can change and then email or discuss the feedback with the changes highlighted in an attachment of an email, especially if the work is urgent. However, if an individual is making the same presentational errors over and over then I would say it is okay to send the work back for them to make the changes as they will become aware & start paying attention to detail especially when the reports will be reported up to higher chain of senior management. In my case, the error occurred once.

My manager was always one to discuss the essence of time management, but I found this to be very hypocritical of him. I have always said to myself that you should always practise what you preach before you expect this from others. His communication was very poor, he would email me back and forth or on teams for changes he needed me to do and would list them but what I have always questioned is, the time you took to type that email is the same amount of time that could have been taken to make the changes especially if they are small. Yes, there is the element that you can learn attention to detail as a skill here but if you are being chased for changes and your manager is aware you are working on another task then the logical sense would be to make the changes as a manager and allow your staff to continue on the work they are doing, especially if they are very focused on it.

This is the first time I have come across a Manager who is one to pass the work around instead of giving a helping hand. Yes, Managers are known for delegating work and being the ones who are responsible for the performance of the team and reviewing work. But a good manager is one who also pitches in to help the team, allowing them to focus on one task as opposed to ten of which two are truly urgent, and one who does not allow their stress to become the stress of the team.

I have openly discussed with my manager that I have anxiety, but it has worsened since I started this role due to the nature of the role being very fast-paced which never gave me time to settle in or understand the tasks I was doing. I love challenges and working under pressure for sure but most importantly I like to also have time to understand why I am doing the tasks so that if I am asked a question, I can answer it confidently. Having been a month, I thought it was fine I would just keep on going and things would click into place and start making sense.

Whilst I had told my manager in my one-month weekly catch-up, that I was not happy with my development and on-boarding due to not being explained tasks or having a neat and clear spreadsheet to work on to understand what was driving certain numbers, I was told I was rushing my learning and just have to trust the process and it would all click into place, there is no pressure. You would assume that when a manager says this, they stick to their words of reassurance.

After this meeting I was quite upset as I was not enjoying my experience. I did not feel heard, and my manager was saying one thing but then rushing and overwhelming me with new tasks which tended to link to the first tasks I had done. Well, if I did not understand why I was doing the first task then I would be slower than he would have expected for the second task.

His words of 'have trust in the process' made no sense, as there was no process because he did not create a process. After mentioning numerous times that tasks need to be explained to me face to face or clearly over teams if I am working from home with an example shown of what you are expecting, my manager carried on continuing teaching me in a way he thought was efficient. But it was not efficient at all, it made no sense. His methods of teaching and training me were not working.

I remember when I first started my manager had mentioned to me that the team was all new and at the beginning he struggled and made lots of mistakes until it got to a point where it was no longer excusable. Furthermore, he had been on the team for eighteen months before he became a manager and knew a lot. Therefore, I questioned myself as to why my mistakes are not excusable when I have only been in the role for a month, and why am I not allowed to work at a slower pace to settle comfortably into my role? The average time to settle in a role is three to six months. Somehow this manager judged me after a month.

At the end of the two-month mark, my manager's attitude became more patronising and I didn't see the point of this at all. Yes, you are a manager, but it does not mean you let the power get to your head or you need to put on a pretence of acting like a manager because you lacked management and leadership skills. I have had many managers in my career, all of whom are not perfect, and neither are we, but they have never put me down or told me I am not good enough.

My three-month probation period was coming up and I was very nervous and scared because the relationship between me and my manager was not great. I knew he would find some excuse to ensure that I either failed my probation or it got extended. The worrying got worse due to the build-up of my meeting, and I began to have migraines. I have always suffered from migraines, but they usually come twice every two weeks, however, in this role my migraines were occurring every three days. The anticipation was killing me.

The more my manager became pushy and spoke to me in a not-so-pleasant manner, I noticed that I did not feel motivated anymore. I wasn't active and began to not care anymore because I was mentally prepped to just quit my job. However, I felt as if this was me running away instead of waiting to hear the outcome of my probation.

It was before the probation meeting day. My manager and the head of the department were on the call and what I expected occurred. I was told that my probation was going to be extended for a further three months because I had not shown them any senior skills or work to suggest otherwise. At this point, I was frustrated because I knew no matter what I said they were not willing to hear me out.

That weekend I began to panic, stopped eating, and began to have too little or excessive sleeping patterns. That continued for a few weeks. My self-confidence was shattered as I had never been in this position before in my life. That following Monday I had no energy to deal with any more bullshit or negativity, smaller tasks began to feel harder or take me longer, and when I was rushed to deliver a deadline, I began to become hot and sweaty. This was all due to how my manager treated me after that meeting. He became very cold and distant. Furthermore, if my on-boarding was done correctly as it was for other new starters then this situation would not have occurred. Not saying that my manager is all wrong; this is not the point I am trying to portray, but he needed management training and learning how to manage staff correctly. I began to feel unvalued and very resentful towards him.

On my way home that Monday, I cried louder and louder and nearly fell asleep behind the wheel because I was mentally fed up. I made a conscious decision to stop going into the office because it made no difference whether I was in the office or not as the communication and trust between me and the manager was tarnished. I felt as if I was his target. I have always believed that it is beneficial to go to the office as you will get to learn from other individuals and have constructive meetings where you can bounce off ideas. In my role, I was not receiving any support from my manager, so I was just better off working from home.

For a moment, I thought I would give my manager the benefit of the doubt and therefore I began to speak with other managers in the finance function with whom I had built a relationship. However, whenever I did mention my manager's name, the feedback I heard was not positive. Everyone mentioned that he is a new young manager, and he has had many confrontations with other managers due to his requests being rude and he came across as very abrupt. This also resulted in others ignoring his requests. This reassured me that I was not the problem because for a while I kept blaming my knowledge and competence in the role.

It had got to a point in time where when I did manage to go into the office, I was called into a meeting room and my manager began to point out the flaws of my work and began to give me negative feedback which had no content or development actions to be taken away from that meeting. He began to say, 'That doesn't look right at all, why did you do that, this can't happen again, how are you going to fix it, how should you have fixed it.' At this point, I spoke back to defend myself. I stated, 'There is no real solution here as I have felt you have always been against me, and you are not the type of manager I want to work with and there is no learning or development that you could offer.' I could see I offended him but at that point, I did not care because his behaviour was not excusable. I then resigned with the hugest sigh of relief before I walked out of the meeting room.

The very next day I emailed Human Resources my resignation letter. I already had a meeting in the diary with them to discuss my experience, but instead, they used that meeting to hear my reasons for leaving in the form of an exit interview. I had mentioned all the reasons above why I cannot cope or manage the workload anymore due to not learning or being taught correctly and patiently and I began to have severe chest pains. Furthermore, I mentioned that my manager failed to remember that I was not someone who came from this industry background so if this was going to be an issue, they should not have hired me because after this experience, I am now very scared to work for this industry and this is something I am still dealing with.

Human Resources was very empathic and told me to sign off that Friday as I was not in the right frame of mind to deal with that sort of stress and anxiety. In a way, I felt they understood that my manager's attitude was not correct and that my on-boarding was not done correctly.

I ended up going on stress leave for a month and did not work during my resignation period as I began to have panic attacks and found it difficult to even talk when I thought about returning to work or facing my manager. I did write an informal grievance to Human Resources on my very last day of work as I thought it was important to get my view across in a professional and written manner. My informal grievance was eleven pages long where I wrote about my experience, what I would have expected, and what outcome I wanted from the grievance. I even went one step further to add a few screenshots to show some of the points I mentioned to them.

Two main things I learned from this job are that it's important to set goals for your staff and then to track them during catchups and discuss any improvements needed to reach the goal but in a supportive manner as well as praise for areas done very well. These goals should be used to help develop skill sets for your staff so that they can grow and be in a better position when it comes to applying for more senior roles. This should not be used to judge or point out flaws if someone does not meet them. Seniors' job is to help staff and allow flexibility, to have open conversations with their employees, so they agree and understand expectations and why goals were set. However, my manager made goals for me without discussing them. He emailed them to me a few weeks before my probation meeting which was not ideal because I would have assumed that this would have been done in the first few weeks in the role, so it was clear what I was working towards.

Furthermore, this company has something called the 'pillars' which are broken down into six or seven skills that a senior needs to have, and then broken into levels, basic, intermediate, and advanced. All seniors are meant to be achieving intermediate however these were never explained to me. In fact, I had to request this after my probation meeting as to why this wasn't shown to me when other new starters who joined around the same time as me were aware of this. Again, this shows that my manager did not fulfil his duties. They were meant to arrange a meeting with me to discuss the pillars, but this never happened as deadlines came before their staff welfare and development. However, their missions and values state otherwise.

When I finally did finish my role in December, I was very broken inside and therefore I began to reflect a lot on what or if I could have done differently. This was important for me because I have always had leadership qualities from a young age and therefore have an expectation of what I would want to be like when I do reach that stage of my life. This experience taught me a lot about how important it is to learn from the good and bad experiences I had and how I was going to use them to make myself a better person.

I cannot stress enough how important it is to send staff on regular courses or even online courses where they can develop themselves. This is a clear example of where my manager who was new to his role, who was struggling, and who had openly admitted this to me and other individuals in the open platform, could have benefitted from management courses. However, he always gave grey area answers as he never knew how to deal with certain situations, even though this is fine as he will learn on the job but it was coming to a year for him so you would expect by now, he would know better.

Since I left, I also found out that another new starter who started two weeks before me had also left due to similar reasons. This is the reassurance I needed weirdly and oddly to know that I was not the sole problem.

Since I left, I have started attending coaching and therapy sessions to work through my self-esteem. I am happy to openly admit this. However I may not have been, a few years back.

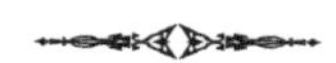

Comparing and Opinion

If we say that we don't compare ourselves or let the opinions of others affect us, then we are delusional. We all in some shape or form let the opinions of others float through our minds or at random moments during the day. At some point, we start to dwell on how we are perceived by others and why they come to that conclusion, and this later makes us believe that we need to change ourselves to be validated or loved. But the truth is, you cannot please everyone and you should not need to. Those who love you will understand you on your good days and bad days. You are allowed to have a crappy day and feel lost and angry. I for one take my anger out on my loved ones. They think I am crazy sometimes, but they love the crazy. We always need that one person who just gets us, for me that is my partner; without judgment or reacting back the same way I feel, he just lets me scream it out.

In my younger years, I never cared about social media or how people viewed me as a person. At school I was always called the teacher's pet, at work, I was called the outspoken one and at home, I am called the funny or over-caring one. Do you see how each group of people views me differently? This may be because of the way I present myself or am, in a different environment. It is fine to be different or tailor yourself to different environments, scenarios, or groups of people but always ensure that you are being yourself. You do not need to change for anyone but for yourself.

Your job is to fight for your happiness and that is your responsibility as no one else will do it for you.

I, for one, have let social media affect my life which has made me very insecure. Up until recently, I have learned how to value myself, my accomplishments, and my goals in life. As I mentioned, we all compare ourselves to others mentally or physically or compete with others by setting benchmarks as an excuse for motivation. I have always worked very hard in my career as an Accountant but then during breaks I began to look at social media to get away from the stress at work. Little did I know, I began to see others having more fun careers or having the time of their life whilst I was working late hours and weekends. This indirectly began to affect my view of life and how I viewed my life in comparison to others. I used to feel a little bit of envy and I would be lying if I said I did not. The secret is, to be honest with yourself about your feelings and take the steps to understand why you feel a certain way and how you are going to change it.

As I got a little older, I began to compare myself to others based on career choices. I began to view people's LinkedIn profiles and saw that people were in higher positions than me or getting promoted within their roles in their company. This started to affect me mentally as I wondered why I was not in the same boat; I was putting in all the hours and doing all my work to the right standard. Furthermore, I felt like a failure and thought there was something wrong with me if I was not getting to where I needed to be.

I began to work extra hard at work and applying for well-recognised companies as I thought this was what would make me feel like I was equal to my old peers or individuals from university. Once I did get my foot through the doors of the big white-collar companies, I worked every hour I could and went over and beyond my role to make a name for myself. I wanted to become established and get recognised in the company so that if there were ever any promotion opportunities I would be considered.

However, this was my biggest flaw and only within the last year or so, I have come to realise that I had wasted so much time focussing on what everyone else was doing rather than what I should be doing in life which brings me fulfilment. I began to notice that I did not need to go hundred miles per hour and I needed to slow down what I was doing because I was just burning myself out and becoming a very unhappy person. Every small thing would get to me before as I was always busy and running around trying to tick things off, but who I was doing this for and why I was doing it began to cross my mind. I was not doing it for myself because if I had, I would not have felt it like a chore or so painful. The companies I worked for enjoyed having a hard worker who was always flexible and working around the clock but whether this was recognised is another question.

I have only been promoted in two of my jobs but that was due to me making myself extra visible by getting my hands stuck in every project. However, did I need to do that to get noticed? If this was the case, then I would have been considered for promotions in my other jobs but did not. Therefore, now that I am in my thirties and reflecting much on my career choices, I have concluded that I do not need to work super hard to be noticed or promoted, I just need to be loyal and focus on producing efficient work as a reliable employee.

When I now look back at all those years, I somewhat feel like they were wasted but I want those who are just starting in their careers or having a career change to focus on the 'why' element. I want you to make decisions with caution and speculate on your choices. Ask yourself why you want to work for the company you have applied for or are currently working at. Are you working there due to the benefits being great or due to the great career progression you will possibly working toward? Are you working there because that will open more doors for your future career goal? But the ultimate and most important question of them all is - are you happy and do you feel fulfilled or will you a few years down the line when you achieve your goal? What will you do next once you reach your goals, if you say that you have reached your end goal and are comfortable remaining there for a few years? Then that is fine but we are complex humans, we always want more or set ourselves challenges to push ourselves.

But for those who have achieved the goals through hard work but have missed out on life for all those months or years, was it worth it? Will you see yourself doing the same work for years to come, because life is short and therefore you need to ensure that time is taken out for yourself and that you are happy doing whatever you are. I find it very hard to define happiness or fulfilment and still to this day I am still discovering what this means. I always thought happiness meant being successful or having lots of money but as I got older, I realised that those were essentials to live but not happiness.

What truly brings me happiness is being around my family, making others feel empowered, and having time for myself. Success on the other hand means I am a better person than I was yesterday or learning from my mistakes because the only person who I should be competing with or comparing myself to, is me. I always have no time to be angry with myself for feeling like I have failed because I am now much more mature to care about who likes or hates me, I have more important things to do. It takes a lot of time and effort to be angry and it's a devotion when you can be devoting it to something more positive. I cannot let the opinions of others during my career define me or make me feel less of a person, instead I have now adopted the mind-set of having more important things to focus on and if those individuals want to be a part of my journey of discovery and growth then be a part of it otherwise, I will just continue my life with or without you.

We will all review the terms happiness and success differently and it's okay to have different definitions. I encourage you to be different because no two people on this earth have the same mind-set. However never compare yourself to others because what we see on social media is all planned or captured after a few tries of trying to perfect a picture or video, be yourself, be different, and be honest with yourself. During recent events, I have come to explore social media in a different light than I did before. As mentioned, before I would feel the need to compare and believe what I saw but now I have learned to not believe everything at face value or assume that what I am seeing is true, because I am not there, I was not present when that moment was captured and most importantly, I am not them. I need to live for myself and do what makes me feel truly valued because no one will remember how many likes I have or how successful I was, but they will remember me by the difference in life I have made to others or what messages I have taught others.

I want to have a guilt-free life going forward and what I mean by this is, I don't want to be happy or successful if it means I am giving a false representation of myself or being someone else to prove my worth to others. I want to have a peaceful life without feeling as if I lied to someone for selfish reasons or to get to the top of the leaderboard. Sharing knowledge, life lessons, and experiences we have had with others is a powerful tool. Not only does it make you feel fulfilled, but it also allows you to stop others from making the same mistakes in a shorter timeframe. Even though it may have taken you ten years to realise or in my case four to five years, it does not mean that I need to watch someone else struggle. However, it's important to change yourself before you decide to go on to change the world or conquer it. You should only advise others if you have been through a similar situation which is relatable but ultimately you need to allow them to take the final step.

We are all indirectly coaches in life, we live through situations, we feel a certain way when a situation presents itself and we act accordingly. Sometimes we are reactive, like I have been in my twenties which is something I am working on. Regardless of how we are, we all have the experiences to go and educate others and advise or recommend action or thought, whether it's right or wrong, it's not for us to judge. The ultimate decision needs to be taken by the seeker of the question as we do not live in their shoes or know their lives or personal commitments. What I ask is, to be open and transparent to help someone in need.

When I was comparing myself to others or the size of my body to those who had my ideal body type, I did not have many people to talk to. It's normal to feel as if you're lacking in something but that only means you have a hole to fill, you need fulfilment. You need to seek the answers for yourself, but the answer does not lie in someone else's life or how you see it. The answer lies much deeper down within you and it's your job to discover it and try different things to identify it. I did those very things. I tried to routine my day to allow myself to find time to do activities, and yet I was comparing myself to others. If it wasn't for my partner just listening to me or supporting me, I do not think I would be where I am today. He was the missing piece of the puzzle who always grounded me and reminded me that I needed to focus on myself and block everyone else out.

I have often let the opinions of others make me feel like I am not good enough. I cannot count the times I have been told that I come across as too bubbly or that I am very transparent and vocal. Hearing these from others in different workplaces gets to the point where you begin to believe that maybe it's true, maybe I am overly friendly, or too vocal at inconvenient times. However, if many people are saying the same things, then you believe that there is some truth to that, and though it may be, you need to just ensure that you listen to it and analyse yourself, but it doesn't mean that you become fake or pretend to be someone else. You can be bubbly with your trusted peers or in meetings but retain the element of professionalism.

Furthermore, you can be vocal and transparent with seniors when asked for feedback but ensure you articulate it in a way from which you are seeking an action to be taken rather than just venting it out to feel better. The choices and words we use are powerful so take your time to act on something or say something because you will be surprised at how small use of words can make all the difference.

This is something I have learned from my reflection and now I am sharing it with you. I have maintained the element of bubbliness as that is me, in general, but I control how much of that is shown, to selective people. This does not mean I am changing myself, but it simply means that I am showing it in small doses in a professional environment in comparison to outside of work.

Furthermore, we have all at some point in our life compared our salary to our peers' or others' we know who work in the same field or role. What does this achieve? It won't change the situation at all. If anything, you will just get yourself worked up in a situation you cannot control. Money is one major factor that drives us because it provides us with the tools we need to survive in life. You should not measure money against your happiness. We all need money to pay our bills and for our holidays, but we should not work in a role that gives us a comfortable life in which money is not a problem because with money comes more responsibility.

You may be earning a lot of money where you are working day and night and trying to always be on top of things at work but then have no time to spend that money. So, ask yourself, who or what exactly are you working so hard for if you don't have the time to spend it or use it for yourself? On the other hand, we have those who are juniors who do not earn as much but work very hard to get established and have the time of their life because they are smart. They know the balance of work and play. They are wise to save a little and then make the time to use the remainder to enjoy life which brings them happiness.

The message here presents itself very clearly, no matter what position you are in a company, you need to ensure your role brings you fulfilment and you want to wake up for work. Secondly, money is not the only reason you are working in your current role. Thirdly, is that you value yourself and understand it is important to recharge yourself and make time for yourself. If that means taking two days off a month or three then so be it. You do not need to have an overseas holiday booked to allow yourself to have those days off. You are the only person who understands yourself and you are the only person who needs to ensure you are happy.

I have now learnt that the opinions of others just gave me strength because even though they are judging me it just shows that they are paying attention to me. Clearly, I am doing something right if they are focused on me as a person and my actions. It's important to be able to listen and reflect, on how much of what is being said is true and if any actions need to be taken to make you stronger and wiser.

This process has taken me time to accept and learn. I used to just feel judged or attacked and always wondered why I was hearing from a third party regarding how people felt about me. Well, if I have not heard it from that person directly then I ignore it because they have not found the time or reason to address it with me directly. For those who directly speak to me about my actions, I respect and admire them because they have seen something in me that I may be biased towards. On the other hand, I have also learned that others just do not want to hurt your feelings so may ask someone else close to us to explain on their behalf. As I mentioned it's your job to reflect and act accordingly.

We all represent ourselves as a brand and therefore we need to present ourselves in a positive and approachable manner because after all we only have one life, and we must live it well. We are here in this world to live and learn and pass it on to others regardless of their age or where they are in life. We are good enough for ourselves and should not let anyone else tell us otherwise. We have the ability to change our bad habits, but we need to do it at a pace that suits us and not one that pleases or is expected from others. You do not need to compare or let the opinions of others define you or change to be someone you were not born to be. You need to find your purpose in life and act accordingly because if you cannot find your purpose or reason for living then no one else will find the answer to the question for you. You need to be a better version of yourself and be a happier person than you were yesterday. However, you need to take risks to see the rewards.

You will only know yourself truly if you know your purpose in life and why you want to fulfil that purpose. Those answers won't be easy to find but that's the beauty of it all. You need to live in this hard world to solve the mystery. There will be bumps along the way but enjoy them and embrace them because each bump has a hidden meaning, your role is to overcome it. The world is always awaiting someone to make a change or solve an issue. We all face for example the cost-of-living crisis or poverty around the world, and you could be that one person who makes the difference. Never doubt yourself or let others say it's impossible because if that were true, I would not be writing this book for you all to read. I will make a change and you are welcome to join me in my journey. You can do it too if you focus on yourself, your happiness, and your purpose because comparing myself and listening to others' negative views of me never did me any good.

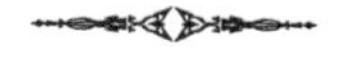

Fear

Fear is a feeling or emotional state of mind that always holds us back from progressing to where we want to be. However, why does fear occur? Usually fear occurs because we initially think that we are not good enough for a job, a person, or for the goals we set. We get ourselves in that mindset that there is no point in trying to work through the fears because you will not achieve what you desire. However, we create these false thoughts in our minds or start feeling negative because not only do we feel that we are not good enough, but we begin to create barriers that put us off.

There are many instances and forms in which fear presents itself. For example, investing in a course that costs thousands of pounds, applying for a job that is one level above our current role, or studying for an exam. However, these negative thoughts stop our productivity and slow us down from achieving our goals. Most successful people have got to where they are because they took risks. Were they scared? Probably but these risks only gave them life lessons of what not to do and what to do better next time. Rewards and results will present themselves, but you need to be able to take that leap of faith, whether that is investing in yourself, which is what I did. I invested thousands of pounds in self-studying ACCA. I was scared, and I kept thinking - why do I need it? I kept finding excuses to not invest in myself by telling myself that others have done it and set up a business without a qualification. It's too much money or I have this or that to do. But these were all excuses. Excuses will only delay your progress and let others achieve their goals because you did not do the research or outline why you need this qualification.

I, for one, needed this qualification as I wanted to teach and coach individuals and show them that if I can do it, anyone can. I could probably set up my own business without the qualification but that just makes it harder as my experience will not be enough to attract clients. It will gain the trust of clients that know what I am doing. Furthermore, I will learn techniques that will benefit me as a coach or tutor myself and also help me see the world differently. I concluded that I needed this qualification because I am learning from those who have done it from the beginning, and they know best what to do and what not to do which saves me time struggling on my own. Investing in yourself is the best asset for yourself and one that no one can take away from you. With this qualification, I can then go on to develop my business in a way that I want but essentially, I will learn the basics of what is needed, something which would take me months to learn if I did it on my own. Time is critical, there are always a million things we need to do in a day but having a plan set in place can not only help you work but also develop yourself.

Furthermore, I have jumped roles during my career and had short-term roles that lasted a few months compared to some gaps on my resume. My fear initially was that by having gaps on my resume it would look bad and show employers that I am not motivated to find another job and I often felt judged at times, when I was asked the question of why I left my previous role. However, there was nothing to be judged about, I just needed to be honest and learn to not take it personally because those individuals were not in my shoes.

My reasons for leaving my previous short-term roles were due to being bullied by my manager and the other, just not being a cultural fit for me as well as jobs not being advertised correctly. However, the lesson here is not to regret it, I needed to learn from my mistakes, and what I learned was that me jumping into another role to avoid having a gap on my resume was not correct. Even though I needed a break, I was better off resigning from my post if I could financially be able to survive a few months whilst finding a correct role.

I let the opinions of recruiters and myself get into my head, and it replayed like a broken record. I kept having the fear that other employers would not want to hire me or that a gap on my resume would show that I was lazy or not active. But then you come to a point where you feel like a failure and a loser for allowing yourself to have a gap on your resume. I felt so negative about the whole gap in my resume situation that I let myself be dragged into a dark hole or applied for roles that matched what I was looking for. I then just accepted it without real thought. However, this has worked out in the past by luck, it will not always work out and this time it did not. Having a gap on my resume felt like the end of the world for me and it's funny how much we overthink things that are not life-threatening situations but they seem so huge in our minds and this only occurs because we let it.

In March 2023, I decided to leave my job, despite being there for only two months, I just knew in my gut that it was not for me. This time I trained my mind to not feel so bad about it. Only you know what's best for you and asking others for their opinion and advice will just increase the confusion or make your stay in the role for a little longer just to make it look good on your resume. I heard from a lot of people to just stay in the role for six months so that it looks good on your resume and then start looking for my ideal role. If I listened to these individuals then I would not be writing this book today and passing on my knowledge and experience. I decided to leave, and it was the best decision I made because I had a realisation that I did not want to be an Accountant anymore but wanted to do something more fulfilling within Accounts.

I have always believed that no experience is wasted in life, it is just a soul-searching experience where you trial and error on what you do and do not like. It always opens doors for you to explore new challenges and make a judgemental call as to whether you want to progress further into that field or try something new. I am currently thirty and I have probably only worked 25% of my career, however, I still have 75% left to work before I can retire, or less if I retire sooner through the success of my career journey. The biggest takeaway from this chapter which I want everyone to reflect on is, are you happy in your role or are you just staying because you are too comfortable and scared to try something in case it does not work out?

If you do not learn to handle risks or failure, then you will always be one to regret your life when you look back and say the one phrase, I despise which is, 'what if'. I no longer have the 'what if' element in my life because it took me nine odd years to accept that it's okay to not be where I am supposed to be or that it's okay. I found my passion late in my life. My goal is to make you all feel valued and reflect on your career choices and happiness. Whether this helps you find your passion or makes you think to help others who have been in my position then I have achieved my purpose.

I am currently unemployed, and I am loving it because I knew for my mental health and for me to heal from the last two bad experiences, I just needed time to myself. It doesn't mean that I needed a fancy holiday or needed to spend lots of money to heal myself but just meant I needed to use my time more productively to find out what and where in my career I want to be and this is something which I could not truly give any thought to whilst I was miserable in my last two roles. Whilst having the time off I have been writing this book to help others understand that there are others out there who feel the same way as them.

I have always wanted to be an entrepreneur, and this is something that I am working towards and hope to achieve within the next few years whilst also finding a role in an educational field to gain more exposure. This does mean that I must take a pay cut and start from the bottom but it's the ultimate decision of whether I want to be in a role I hate or in a role I enjoy in which the money and benefits will come along in the future. I want my job to not feel like a job but a hobby. Being patient is vital, results will not come straight away and you need to be able to accept this. The reason I want to work towards becoming an entrepreneur is because I am an individual who wants to operate and teach others my knowledge and experiences in my own way and have full control as well as flexibility. If this is you, then take the time to explore your options or try doing it part-time to see if it will work out and if it doesn't, it's fine. Just re-map your goals and try another strategy. Failure only makes us stronger as humans and it leads us to think outside the mediocre mindset which leads to amazing new opportunities.

Another factor that also plays on my mind is that the world is now becoming very dominated by technology and in the future, roles will be reduced due to robotics taking over and finding quicker and more efficient ways of working. Although this sounds very sceptical, I have seen some of my previous employees not hiring as many roles as they used to because companies now invest in new programmes or IT data systems which carry out the role that an employee previously did. This is one fear which always creeps into my mind because I am an individual who thinks about my life in the long term rather than the short term when it comes to my career. As I have previously mentioned, this can be very bad for one's mental health as you should live in the moment, but you also need to have plans in place if things do not work out, for contingency.

I have read many articles and heard testimonies of individuals who hate their job and that is the cold hard truth. I have seen people walk into work with fake smiles, who are miserable whilst working, and just keep drinking coffee to take a break from their screen or to pass the time. I was one of them because I was afraid to listen to my gut and passion. Whilst being an employee I learned what it truly meant to be an employee and that was having no leverage, listening to your boss and that their way is correct, listening to the wrong people, being very closed-minded, and having my confidence shut down if I spoke up. Whilst I am now looking for roles in a field I enjoy, I will ensure that it is a right cultural fit for me as an employee because if it means I must become a 'yes' person without my opinion or feedback being valued then I rather just work towards the goal of being an entrepreneur without having a job in the background.

However, being an entrepreneur will mean that I will be more positive, and open-minded, helping others find solutions to their problems and having the flexibility to also focus on myself and that will come with its challenges, but I am ready to embrace them. This in my eyes will be my perfect job and whilst many of us define a perfect job in different ways, a perfect job for me will mean having no alarm clock, no discrimination, no work politics, no boss, and no fake small talk.

Whilst having the perfect job can seem like it's impossible, you can have this if you devote time and effort to setting up your own business. However, you need to ensure that you do not burn out to make it successful. Your first initial step will be to begin setting up the business which would include your content, legalities, and learning how to attract clients. From those clients, their testimony and recommendations will boost your business as well as your marketing. This is something I will achieve within a few years because the perfect business for me will mean having unlimited income potential, having a meaningful business, and time freedom. You can also achieve this if you trust yourself. Nothing is impossible in this world, it's our fear and mindset that makes it feel that it's a fantasy and a dream that will never be a reality.

Whilst many of us are scared to leave our current roles to start a new adventure, there are others out there who have been in our shoes and succeeded. If you are a person who is worried or scared like I was a few months ago then stay in your role if you can mentally handle it whilst launching your business and when it gets to a stage where you are happy and meet your financial goals, then quit your job. As mentioned, we all need stability, and it's vital for our survival but we all have different commitments and financial difficulties but you need to decide when it's the best time for you to start your new journey, no one will tell you or help you to get there.

For many months, whilst I have been launching my business in the background, I did get anxious and stressed out because I kept having the odd thought of why someone would want to be coached by me and, am I good enough? But these thoughts just led me to invest myself and now all my internal thoughts get answered by a coach who was once in my position and helps me to trust myself. From today onwards, I want you to see me as a coach. My job is to guide you and help you reflect on your career, life choices, and goals. However, my role is not to give you the answers. You need to find qualities within yourself that remind you that you are good enough and that you will be successful, not if you will be but when you will be. Choosing the right words will also change your mindset and motivate you to achieve your goals.

Fear is a feeling that we cannot just erase, run from, or block out. We need to embrace the fear and let it sit there for thirty minutes or so but after that, we need to move on and focus on our purpose. The more time and effort we put into achieving the goal the more fear will reduce itself because you can look back to how much you have done. I use fear or anger as motivation. As odd as it sounds it motivates me to push myself or to set a benchmark for myself to prove that I can do it.

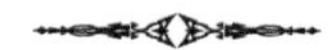

Needing Help

It is always hard to admit we need help or hard to believe that it is needed. It got to a stage in my life when I knew something was not sitting right with me and that I bottled up all my emotions or sugar-coated how I felt. We are brought up with the perception that we need to show our strong sides to individuals and cannot show our weaknesses. Although I do believe this at times as I have had many people take advantage of my weaknesses when I just needed support, I have learned that if I feel vulnerable or have a moment of weakness, I need to just let it out. Those individuals who are not there for you when you need them or mock you are not your friends or colleagues. You need to distance yourself from those toxic people. Even though the word 'toxic' sounds very harsh, it is the truth.

Since having two bad experiences in my career, I began to have suicidal thoughts because I felt like a failure, a loser, and incompetent to do anything in life. Even though the thoughts in my mind were telling me to keep on going and trying to find a job in which my passion lies, my body was telling me otherwise. I began to have horrible sleeping patterns where I would fight to stay awake because I wanted to feel drained in the morning and just stay in bed to avoid my family and the public.

I began to ignore my true friends and pretend that I never saw their messages or calls. Furthermore, I stopped any physical exercise I was doing, one of which was taking my dog for a walk. I stopped eating because I did not feel hungry and knowing that I did not eat much, my body felt as if it had. I began to have self-harming thoughts again because that was the only thing I knew I was good at to release the pain; however, I did not carry out this action because I knew the scars once they healed would not be worth it. I would even not shower for a day or two because I felt like I had no energy and just wanted to be left alone with my thoughts. I needed to heal myself, but I just did not want to accept it.

My mind felt that if I sought help then I would feel more insecure about myself and that it would be embarrassing if I ever mentioned it to anyone. One issue that I noticed was that my anger got bad, and I began to become short-tempered about any little things. If I felt as if I was not heard by people or that I was interrupted when I finally found the energy to talk, I would just see red. My anger would jshoot to a hundred and I did not realise how bad it was until I began to see my family and my partner point it out.

Although they would laugh it off and try to calm me down, it just made the whole situation in my head a whole lot worse. The worst thing you can do is tell someone to calm down when they are angry. This is something that I have learned through my own experience of being angry and from those I have tried to calm down in the past. The best thing you can do is just hear the individual out without interrupting them and let them vent. There are always awkward situations where this is done in public and it might not sit well with you to display a public show. However, in those instances just ask the individual to move to a more discreet place and to lower their tone so that you can understand their point of view.

My partner began telling me to lower my tone because he was unable to have a conversation with me with all the shouting I was doing. However, he would say it calmly with a smile without reacting to my behaviour. He set an example of how I should explain my anger more appropriately if I want to be heard and now and then he would smile or try to make me laugh to lighten the mood. While this worked for me it was a short-term fix.

You are allowed to be angry for a moment or two. However it's a skill that we all need to reflect on after the event has passed. You need to ask yourself, could you have handled it differently, spoken in a more adult manner to get your view across and could you have possibly addressed it at a different point in time rather than there and then? This is something that I know seems so much easier to reflect on and say, 'Ah, I do this already', but if you are doing it already then why is your behaviour when you are angry not changing, and why is it not appreciated by people.

We all need to scream and shout in moments in life because I will be the first to admit, it's hard to hold back your first initial thoughts and reaction. We never plan for our lives to take these unfortunate turns, but it happens. Scream and shout but in a private place. I have screamed against my pillow, in a forest, or in the shower and it has felt amazing and taken a load off my shoulder but again this was a temporary fix.

As hard as it was for me to admit to my anger issues and write about it for the whole world to know one side of me, it's necessary for me to let others know that I am there for them and that I am also like them.

I decided that I needed help and no one else was going to do it for me. I called my GP one day and told them that I felt very low and felt as if I was a danger to myself. They decided to direct me to therapy. I waited a few days to get a slot to be seen and it made me very anxious and stressed. I began to think about why I just admitted that to my GP and do I want the help? I decided that if I did receive a call, I was going to ignore it and just pretend it was a mistake. My head could not comprehend all the judgment and questions that I was going to be asked but again this was all in my head. I was always assuming the worst before even giving therapy a go.

The day came when I got a call from the emergency helpline service, and it was surprisingly pleasant. I was asked to discuss my situation and symptoms. They were very active listeners which made me feel more relaxed. I felt as though I was able to have a conversation with them because it was someone with whom I did not need to present my face on camera or meet in person. This led me to feel as though no judgment would be passed as their view would not be biased.

After having a round of questions asked and then scaling up my answers between one to ten, they were able to identify what further help may be needed. However, this was not discussed on the initial call. I was told that I would receive another call in a few days to discuss how I was feeling on a different day to ensure that these feelings were occurring more regularly as opposed to a one-off event. I patiently waited a few days but then began to become a little helpless and hopeless. I just had a feeling that they would delay the process and not contact me back. Again, this was me creating mini-negative scenarios in my mind of what would happen, but I was just causing more harm to myself than good. I know I was looking at the whole situation negatively.

My mind was racing, and I had thousands of thoughts that were driving me crazy and made me feel even more drained. I knew that I needed to get myself together. I began to realise after weeks and months of feeling like a failure that by me having pity on myself or hoping that someone would come to pick up the pieces and rescue me was a fantasy. Whilst awaiting a catch-up call from the emergency helpline services, I decided to find a coach. My friend recommended one to me a few weeks which led me to take my first step of self-healing by applying for a coach to help me through some of my personal issues.

This is a service that offers your six free sessions which last forty-five minutes each and are conducted via a telephone call. You are assigned one coach or two depending on availability and is only for women under thirty. I thought this would be good for me because even though it may have been a situation where I was able to just talk and be heard by someone without feeling afraid of judgment, it was enough for me.

However, the session took me by surprise. I had my first call where I thought a coach was one who would give you solutions and answers, but on that day, I truly learned the meaning of a coach. A coach is someone who guides you to make your own decisions. Their role is to ask you questions that help you think deeper. Even though these questions are simple, we as humans tend to not reflect on more simplistic questions, we need to ask ourselves to answer our questions. We tend to answer our questions in a biased way in which we are not being realistic about the dilemma we are tackling, and we begin to act as if nothing was our fault and others are to blame. If you truly want to help yourself, you need to start being honest and be able to look at yourself in the mirror and accept the truth.

During my first session, I sat in front of the mirror and decided that I was going to be truthful in all the questions asked.

The session started with me explaining why I needed coaching and how I believed it would benefit me. My first session discussed how I felt confused by my career due to the bad experiences I had and how I let it affect me mentally. I put my wealth above my health in my early career which just made me resent myself. I became that very person I did not want to be which was a miserable and lost person.

The session then took a turn where the coach would ask me questions accordingly based on what she was hearing. Surprisingly, this made me think on a deeper level of whether my feeling of failure was truly the issue I was facing or was it something else? This thought remained with me for a few days until I awaited to book my next session. What I mostly liked about this service was that you were able to book your next sessions as and when you needed by simply messaging your coach. Furthermore, you did not need to address one issue in the call but could discuss more than one. I based my coaching sessions on my career because that is where I needed to discover my purpose more but also, I needed closure.

A week later, I received a call from the emergency helpline service to have my catch-up call. The routine was the same where I was asked a series of questions which I had to answer against a rating. At the end of the call, we addressed my symptoms. I was told they were concerned about my well-being as my symptoms showed that I was going through a lot. Even though I have had suicidal thoughts and self-harming but not carried them out, it is still alarming in case things get worse that I would reciprocate my actions.

I decided then I needed therapy for my anxiety and depression and as hard as it was to hear, it felt like a breath of fresh air. I was finally going to address my underlying emotions and feelings with someone who was going to provide me with tools and methods to help me. I knew this was just the beginning, the real work begins when you start applying what you are being taught into practice. As I have mentioned several times in this book, you need to be able to look after yourself because no one else will do it for you. I for one took the first step which was admitting that I needed help for myself and that alone is a hard pill to swallow.

Despite not telling anyone about me having these thoughts except for my partner, it is now my responsibility to heal myself. You do not need to put a timer on how long you must heal. This is a natural process and time does heal a person, but the magic lies in what actions you take to get to that stage. Most of us just assume that the problem will unravel itself after the first or second session of coaching or therapy and that it's not helping. This only means that you have accepted defeat already. The first and second session are just the beginning of your journey and a platform for you to speak and be understood by your therapist. Future sessions are where you will begin to see things from a different perspective and therefore it is important to trust the professionals. Although others may have had a different experience in comparison to me it just means that you need to try a different therapist or find a different service to help you. Help is out there for you as a starting point, but you need to seek it.

I am currently on the waiting list awaiting therapy for my anxiety and depression and it is something that is not in my control. However, what I can do to ensure that I am motivating myself is to create a little routine. Yes, this is a very disciplined routine that can be hard to follow or commit to yourself but all you need to do is have a plan of what you would like to achieve. This is similar to setting goals in which if you do not achieve your goal at a point in time when it can always be moved or delayed, it does not mean that you will not achieve it.

I began by making a list of things that I wanted to do, and one which would bring me happiness. I decided that I wanted to work out and be more physically fit, bake more, and focus on my skincare. I began to start working out at home for ten to twenty minutes which was then followed by ten to fifteen minutes of yoga. I also made it a commitment to take my dog for a long walk every day. I found it very difficult at the beginning to even do five minutes of exercise but it's the sense of completing something no matter how short which made me feel very good about myself.

Also enjoyed the pain I felt after a workout as I knew my body was working hard.

The point here is that it is difficult to say you want to achieve something and then go ahead to do it, but you just need to be able to take baby steps. If you achieve ten out of the twenty-minute workout, it's okay. It's a goal you are working towards so do not be hard on yourself or beat yourself up about it, you will get there.

As much as we hear that breathing is relaxing and calms us down most majority of us will feel like it does not help. I tried it and it never worked for me. However, doing a few breathing exercises by incorporating them in the form of yoga has helped me to feel motivated in the morning. I learned that I was breathing a lot from my chest area so kept all the tension there and was not allowing my body to relax. I began to watch free YouTube tutorials and learned to breathe from the lower abdomen and then work my way up, this also helped with my anger issues.

I have had four anger management sessions via teams and have met some amazing women who are also feeling the same way as me. Although, not everyone shares their reasons for being there, having other individuals within the session made me feel as if I was not alone. During the anger management session, we were taught how we may look at certain situations in different ways, models to try and test, and to keep an anger management log.

I was very sceptical regarding the anger management log because I thought why do I need to do this when I just now am always angry? I gave it a go just like anything you should do in life, and I began to realise what situations and who triggered my anger. This was the light I needed to be shown. Small things just as someone being in the wrong lane but then trying to cut me up made me angry because I saw the world in a black-or-white way. Now I ask myself why I am even reacting. If someone goes in front of me it does not matter because, at the end of the day, we are going in the same direction. So, why am I working myself up about the situation as I am just upsetting myself unnecessarily?

My anger management coach is one who I have the utmost respect for because he just says things as they are without being too sensitive to what he is saying, and we all enjoy that aspect of the therapy. He is humble, and funny and kept it engaging rather than just talking at us without anything going into my mind. Worksheets are provided at the end of each session, and it was my responsibility to read them and try the methodologies or techniques that he suggested. But you need to prepare yourself mentally to be able to understand what the takeaway points from the session were and what steps you are going to try before your next session.

The hard work is done by you at the end of each session because essentially you are reflecting. We all shy away from it, but things don't heal themselves, they heal because you put in the work to get to a happier place.

I currently have finished my anger management classes and this is an experience that I will cherish. I now have the tools that I need to keep practising and incorporating into my everyday life to better myself. I will not put a timeline to my growth, it's a natural process and I am going to embrace it. My biggest achievement in my life is admitting that I needed help and working towards focusing on my well-being as well as putting myself first.

I have been focusing on becoming a better version of myself and I will always shed layers to peel off to get to the core, but I am going to trust myself to hold myself accountable to this. I have also made a chart to write down what went well or bad in my day and then focus on what did not go well by collecting the evidence mentally to understand why I may not have reacted correctly or reciprocated the message someone was trying to get across to me well. I then turn to my anger management worksheet to find a way to ensure if I am put in the situation again, how I will tackle it better.

I appreciate this new version of me, and I am so excited to see what my future holds because my dark times are over, and I have experienced a lot for my age. I am grateful for the opinions of others which just motivated me even more, the obstacles that slowed down my growth, and the rejections I got because I would not be where I am today. The younger version of me would not have understood what I was going through but this version of me now is very thankful. Failure just made me stronger and stronger, and I will build a brand around me where toxic people will not be allowed to enter the world of happiness that I have created. I am good enough for myself and no one else can ever tell me otherwise.

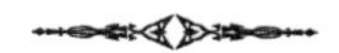

Acceptance

After a year of bad experiences, I have come to terms that I am confused about what I want in my career and where I want to end up. It's okay that I feel this way and for anyone else who also feels the same way. We all have great ambitions that change throughout our lives, and it may feel like we failed because we did not complete what we may have set out to do months or years ago but you have not failed, you have just grown to make better decisions which suit you at that moment in your life. You have also matured and learned that you may have more to explore.

After leaving my last employer I decided that I just wanted a career break, and you can do this at any moment in your life, and don't let anyone tell you otherwise. Therefore, the career break helped me to see the working environment from all angles. I decided that I wanted to use my time wisely by participating in voluntary work which I am still applying for, travelling, and writing this book. I have a dream to open my own coaching and mentoring business to help others but that will be a long-term project which I will continue to work on.

You are allowed to take time for yourself, and you need to as it helps you process the past and makes you think with a clearer head. Yes, you need money to be able to take a career break and have the financials sorted but you can also apply for job seekers or other benefits which you are entitled to for all your past hard work.

After having a few months to myself I have now learned that I do not want to work in a pure accounting role because it was not a fulfilling role in which I felt valuable or enjoyed. I just worked in Accounts because I had a degree in the subject, and it paid well for me to live comfortably. I have now come to terms that my personality needs to be reflected in the next job that I do. I am a bubbly and enthusiastic person who lives to challenge herself and sitting at a desk for most of my life just won't cut it for me, this is not my purpose.

I have heard a lot of opinions from my friends and family that I am wasting my ACCA or degree and I should just continue in my accounting role and work my way up. However, this is just their opinion, it has no reflection of how I feel and therefore I gladly ignored it. You cannot let the opinions of others dictate your life; you need to decide for yourself as you are the person who must continue that lifestyle for years to come. Life is short and if it has taught me anything, it is that it is never too late to have a career change or just to explore something different.

I now embark on a new journey in which I want to explore the world of being a tutor in accounts as I have always liked the interactive side of that role. It will be hard work and long hours, but I am sure that it will be one that I enjoy. The worst-case scenario would be that I won't enjoy it but that's okay because this is the exploring stage for me, I will always wonder 'what if' or assume I know the life of a tutor when I rather judge it for myself.

Becoming a coach and mentor will always be my life goal because we have so much going on in the world that people just need someone to talk to. I have always known that I enjoyed advising and listening to people. I like having conversations that allow individuals to explore their thoughts in more detail because we always find excuses to not give deep thought to important decisions in our lives. For example, I have had friends accept roles just because it was the only offer they had but that's not to say that if they were patient they would have found one that they enjoyed. It's all about knowing yourself and trying to make selective decisions that work for you.

Everyone's situations and circumstances are different, and I respect that but this book is my experience and wisdom I have learned based on my lifestyle. I want you to reflect on the areas which apply to you and to do some soul searching of where in your life you can make changes or which areas relate to you in which you want to act and start making changes. One thing that you do not want to do is live a life because you just need to live. Your work is the foundation that provides you income but also affects your social life, health, time with family, and mental health. These are the main reasons we live or why I live. I want to see my family grow and I want to explore the world without feeling like I need to rush to tick things off my bucket list. You need to live the experience and not just do the experience. If you enjoy your job along the way, it will make a huge difference in how your life is shaped.

If you are at the start of your career or find yourself in a job that you are not entirely happy with then remember that every stop along the way is an opportunity to learn and grow. Every experience no matter how big or small plays a role in shaping who you are and what you can achieve. Never look back and think that the experience you gained was a waste because it wasn't: it just taught you that you are seeking something else and we won't know this until we try new things.

Acceptance is even harder, and we often fall into the trap of always blaming ourselves when things go wrong or don't work out but what good does this do? Accept the areas in which you could have done better or put in more effort and move on. Focussing on creating a better and happier version of yourself is where time should be spent. Don't fall into the trap of feeling sorry for yourself and letting your mind stop you from using that energy or feeling to do something more productive and motivational. I know this is easier said than done but you just need to practise and train yourself to use your time efficiently.

This is the best thing that I have ever done for myself, taking a break from my career and just focusing my energy on other areas in my life that are important for me to focus on to get myself to a happy stage. For me, this included booking a trip to the Cayman Islands to see my friend and just having a moment for myself and my thoughts whilst away from my comfort zone. This helped me to reflect on my life and see things from a different perspective. Seeing the lifestyle in another country opens your eyes to see how everyone in different parts of the country have their own benefits but struggles too. Whilst I was sitting on the beach, I was able to make a mental list of things that I wanted to do differently when I returned to the UK and how I was going to approach them.

The first thought that came to my mind was to focus on finding a job that fitted my needs and wants, even if this meant I needed to compromise a small portion of what I wanted. I would be okay to do this. I made a list of the types of roles and companies I wanted to work for and why. I then mapped out where I was going to apply first and ensured that I asked questions to understand the roles completely before jumping into the role.

The second thought that came to my mind was finding the balance in my life and how I was going to achieve this. This included going out on the weekends with those I wanted to be around and trying different foods and activities that I had not done before. Finding a balance can be hard but not impossible if you start to make it a routine. As I mentioned, we have deadlines to complete but at the end of the day you are required to work your contracted hours, and everything after that is eating up your own personal time. At times we must do longer hours and it's okay but not to the point where you are doing it every day and every week. You will lose yourself in your work and look back to see that you could have done so much more in your life rather than stressing about the work pressure.

Sometimes when we go out shopping, we tend to just spend our money which at the end of the day builds up to a large sum but we enjoy the day. However, some of us spend our money wisely and purchase what we need at that moment in time rather than what we want, as a want can always be completed at a later point in time. However, if we can make strategic decisions when it comes to shopping or spending our money then what is stopping you from making strategic decisions about your life goals and career path. This is due to us not taking the time to focus on ourselves and our long-term plan for the months ahead which will bring us happiness. Instead, we work, work, work, and then come home and complain we are unhappy or end up being moody just to repeat it. However, if you work in a role where you are happy, and management treats you equally and with respect then it becomes a place where you feel valued and see that your input is being listened to. Then work doesn't feel like work on most days but feels like you are going to work on something you enjoy.

I used to get anxious on Sundays, dreading work for the new week ahead. I used to feel as though the weekend went too fast and I was not able to switch off from work, but I have learned this was because I really hated my role and was constantly worrying. This feeling differs for individuals, some just want a longer holiday, a break, or want to relax before another hectic week but you would not be feeling very low if you enjoyed your role.

You need to remind yourself that you are good enough and you haven't come this far by not being good enough. You are perfectly normal if you feel confused in life, career, or just in general about your next steps. You are perfectly normal if you want to have a career change and explore other areas in your field or a different field.

Up until this stage in my life, I still feel scared and anxious about how my life will map itself out but that's also normal. There is a lot of uncertainty in the world, and we just need to educate ourselves about these changes and adjust our plans to fit around them. Nothing is impossible but you need to make it possible by taking action and being a problem solver. Every decision will have risks and rewards. Be scared, be anxious, and be proud of yourself for even considering taking these actions because most of us just sit on the fence hoping for better days. Better days come to those who make them.

Accept that you are living in a world that is becoming very challenging and tough. Rise to the challenge and make it work for you because I believe you can and now you need to.

Be honest in accepting that you are a simple number on the payroll system and are replaceable. So, if there is something you really want to try or dream of doing, do it now or plan it for the months ahead, but do not sit on that thought. The future is uncertain, and you do not want to live with regret that you did not do something for yourself. Your needs and wants are just as important as any company's mission statement and strategic goals.

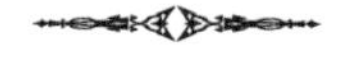

Milton Keynes UK
Ingram Content Group UK Ltd.
UKHW011543310124
437030UK00001B/9